Practical Ultrasound

In the hands of a skilled operator, ultrasound scanning is a simple and easy procedure. However, reaching that level of proficiency can be a long and tedious process. Commended by the British Medical Association, *Practical Ultrasound*, Third Edition incorporates up-to-date techniques and protocols, focusing on the scans regularly encountered in a busy ultrasound department. This book provides everything novice practitioners need to know to become competent and skilled in scanning.

Beginning with the general principles of ultrasound scanning and a guide to using the ultrasound machine, this book provides clear instructions on how to perform scans supplemented by high-quality images and handy tips. Organized according to anatomical site, the chapters include a review section on useful anatomy, scan protocol presented step by step, and a section on common pathology. Maintaining the popular format of the first and second editions, each chapter contains examples of common and clinically relevant pathologies and notes on the salient features of these conditions.

The authors' precise approach puts an immense amount of knowledge within easy reach, making it an ideal aid for learning the practicalities of ultrasound.

Key Features:

- Follows an appealing organization of chapters, developing fundamental knowledge of how to operate the ultrasound machine before moving on to the practicalities of how to scan each anatomical area.
- Presents comprehensive, authoritative, and up-to-date text, integrating anatomical knowledge, practical tips from experts, and common clinical pathologies that are important to recognize.
- Incorporates high-quality ultrasound images with corresponding line drawings indicating the key points to spot.
- Arms you with the practical knowledge you will need when you pick up the ultrasound probe and start out on your own journey of learning the skill of ultrasonography.

Practical Ultrasound: An Illustrated Guide

Third Edition

Dr Jane Alty MB BChir MA(Cantab.) MD FRCP(UK) FRACP

Associate Professor of Neurology, College of Health and Medicine, University of Tasmania, Australia
Consultant Neurologist, Royal Hobart Hospital, Tasmania, Australia

Dr Edward Hoey MBBCh BAO MRCP FRCR

Consultant Cardiothoracic Radiologist
University Hospitals Birmingham NHS Trust, UK

Dr Michael Weston MB ChB MRCP FRCR

Consultant Radiologist (retired), Leeds Teaching Hospitals NHS trust

With collaboration from:

Mr Stephen Wolstenhulme MHSc DMU DCR(R) FHEA
Lecturer in Diagnostic Imaging, University of Leeds
Advanced Practitioner Radiographer, Leeds Teaching Hospitals NHS Trust

Dr Fiona Canavan MB BChir MRCP FRCR
Radiology Specialist Registrar
North Wales, Betsi Cadwaladr University Health Board

Dr Harun Gupta MD DNB MRCP FRCR
Consultant Musculoskeletal Radiologist
Leeds Teaching Hospitals NHS Trust

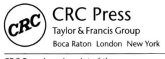

CRC Press
Taylor & Francis Group
Boca Raton London New York

CRC Press is an imprint of the
Taylor & Francis Group, an **informa** business

Third edition published 2025
by CRC Press
2385 NW Executive Center Drive, Suite 320, Boca Raton FL 33431

and by CRC Press
4 Park Square, Milton Park, Abingdon, Oxon, OX14 4RN

CRC Press is an imprint of Taylor & Francis Group, LLC

© 2025 Jane Alty, Edward Hoey and Michael Weston

First edition published by CRC Press 2006
Second edition published by CRC Press 2014

ISBN: 9781032464343 (hbk)
ISBN: 9781032464312 (pbk)
ISBN: 9781003381655 (ebk)

DOI: 10.1201/9781003381655

Typeset in Gill Sans
by codeMantra

Dedicated to the memory of Dr Donal Deery

Contents

Foreword

As predicted in my Foreword to the first edition, this illustrated guide to practical ultrasound has proved to be of tremendous value to ultrasound trainees. Accordingly, the publishers requested a third edition with updates and additions to all chapters.

The demand for ultrasound imaging continues to increase, as does the need for trained operators, and I have absolutely no doubt that this book will continue to be a great help to aspiring ultrasonographers, whether radiographers, radiologists, or trainees from other clinical disciplines.

Dr Henry C Irving
Retired Consultant Radiologist
Previously at Leeds Teaching Hospitals NHS Trust
Past President of British Medical Ultrasound Society

Preface

It is pleasing to see the ongoing enthusiasm for the straightforward step-by-step approach that *Practical Ultrasound* brings and to be invited to write a third edition of this bestselling book. We have received positive feedback from ultrasonographers and radiology trainees all over the world since we first wrote the book. Most often, trainees write to us to explain that this book helped them learn the basics of ultrasound – it gave them direction and a 'recipe' to follow when stepping out on the journey of learning the skills required to become competent. However, some of the readers spotted areas that could be explained better and we have taken this constructive feedback on board when writing the Third Edition of *Practical Ultrasound*. In this new edition, we have refined sections to bring them up to date with current recommendations, reduced some sections that repeated the same information, and also added new clearer images of pathology.

This book has met its original aims to equip the trainee with the skills and knowledge required to start out in the world of ultrasonography, but we also recognize that to become confident and a truly skilled operator, the trainee needs to practice and gain feedback from mentors. We hope this book continues to inspire and support that lifelong path of learning.

About the authors

A/Prof Jane Alty MB Bchir MA(Cantab.) FRCP FRACP MD
Associate Professor of Neurology, University of Tasmania, Australia
Consultant Neurologist, Royal Hobart Hospital, Australia

A/Prof Alty initially trained as a Radiology registrar at the Leeds Teaching Hospital NHS Trust in the United Kingdom before completing specialist physician training as a Neurologist. She moved to Australia in 2019 to take up an academic neurology position and her research involves developing digital biomarkers for neurodegenerative disorders.

Dr Edward Hoey MBBCh BAO, MRCP(UK)
Consultant Radiologist, University Hospitals Birmingham, UK

Dr Hoey is a Consultant Radiologist at one of the largest teaching hospitals in the United Kingdom. He underwent specialist training in Radiology at Leeds Teaching Hospitals and at Papworth Hospital in Cambridge. He is an Honorary Senior Lecturer at the University of Birmingham Medical School and remains active in teaching and research with over 50 peer-reviewed publications. His specialist interests are in Thoracic and Cardiovascular Imaging.

Dr Michael Weston MB ChB MRCP FRCR
Consultant Radiologist, St James's University Hospital, Leeds, UK (retired).

Dr Weston worked as a Consultant Radiologist, with a specialist interest in ultrasound, at Leeds Teaching Hospital NHS Trust in the United Kingdom between 1994 and 2020. His expertise is highly sought, and he has given 257 invited lectures at national and international meetings and conferences. He was the Editor of the *Clinical Radiology* journal between 2018 and 2022 and also an author of *Clinical Ultrasound* 3rd Edition. Eds Paul Allan, Grant Baxter and Michael Weston, Churchill Livingstone, London 2011.

General principles of ultrasound scanning

Optimizing the quality of your ultrasound scan images will increase the information you can obtain from them. Here are some suggestions to help improve image quality and some advice on how to prevent repetitive strain injury (RSI)/work-related upper-limb disorder (WRULD).

1 Ensure the correct orientation of the probe head. One designated end (marked on some probes with a ridge or light) should point towards the patient's head when scanning in the LS (longitudinal/coronal) plane, then, on turning 90° anticlockwise into a TS (transverse/axial) plane, this end will be pointing towards the patient's right side.

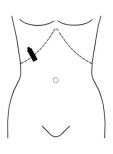
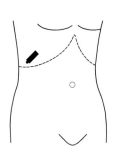
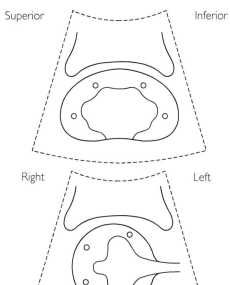

Superior — Inferior

Right — Left

Hint: Running a finger along the probe face will produce a faint ripple on the screen, and it will be obvious which is the correct way round! There is a control that will reverse the image on the screen if you prefer not to turn the probe round (stops the cable from becoming twisted and damaged).

2 Always scan completely off structures to avoid missing pathology at the peripheries e.g., for kidneys, scan completely through and beyond in both LS and TS planes.

3 Scan through an acoustic window whenever possible – e.g. through a full bladder for transabdominal pelvic scans.

4 When examining a cystic lesion, look for features to help characterize it as benign or potentially malignant:

Benign features:
- smooth edge
- thin wall
- echo-free contents
- postacoustic enhancement

Malignant features:
- irregular edge
- thick wall
- internal echoes/thick septations
- poor beam through transmission
- internal blood flow

5 Often malignant changes can be subtle. One tip is to look for 'mass effect', whereby malignant lesions cause distortion of the normal anatomical architecture – e.g. liver metastases often distort the hepatic and portal venous anatomy.

6 Make use of colour Doppler to help distinguish vessels from other structures – e.g. common bile duct versus portal vein/hepatic artery.

DOI: 10.1201/9781003381655-1

7 Use the mnemonic 'PLiSK' when comparing the echogenicity of the abdominal organs. The pancreas is normally more echo-bright than the *liver*, which in turn is slightly brighter than the **s**pleen, which is brighter than the cortex of the **k**idneys. PLiSK is an easy way of remembering the correct sequence and will alert you to the presence of some pathologies – e.g. fatty liver, which appears much brighter than it should (see later).

P LiS K

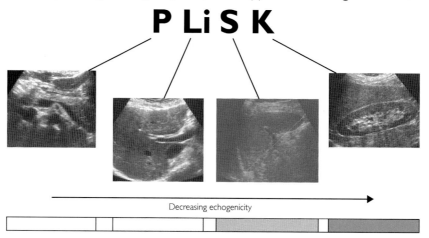

Decreasing echogenicity

8 Measure blood vessel calibre in TS with the probe perpendicular to the vessel long axis; measure from inside of wall to inside of wall. The vessel needs to be assessed in both TS and LS in order to obtain the best TS section and hence the most reproducible measurement.

9 If bowel gas is obscuring a structure, instruct the patient to 'push out stomach', re-examine them later after moving the patient or give a waterload to fill the stomach which will act as an acoustic window.

10 When viewing abnormalities in a fluid-filled structure (e.g. gallstones), always try to obtain images after the patient has changed position. This helps distinguish lesions fixed to a wall (e.g. polyps) from mobile ones (e.g. stones).

11 Always consider patient safety. The mechanical index (MI), which is a measure of tissue effects from ultrasound, should be kept to the lowest level that allows an image to be achieved. Regulations allow MIs up to a maximum of 0.9.

PREVENTING RSI/WRULD

This is a common problem among healthcare professionals who use ultrasound on a regular basis. It most often affects the upper limb of the scan arm and is thought to be caused by a combination of awkward posture due to poor workstation set-up and excessive twisting and pressure on the probe. The following measures will help to alleviate this problem:

- Aim for a mixed caseload during the scan session.
- Adjust the bed height in order to avoid stretching excessively up or down during the scan – have your eyes level with the top of the monitor to avoid excessive neck movements.
- Maintain good seated posture (ergonomically designed stools can help) and consider standing to assess the left kidney or during transvaginal scans.
- Keep close to the patient in order to avoid over-abduction of your arm and rest the elbow of your scan arm gently on the patient.
- Move the patient into oblique/decubitus positions when examining the liver, kidneys or spleen. This prevents excessive rotation of the forearm.
- Apply only light skin pressure with the probe.
- Remember to stretch and to take regular rest periods between patients.
- Consider standing to assess the left kidney or when doing transvaginal scans.
- Consider scanning both left- and right-handed during the day.

2 Using the ultrasound machine

1 Confirm the patient's name, date of birth and address.
2 Explain the nature of the examination and confirm patient consent.
3 Enter the patient's details into the machine (usually via a 'patient data button'). If using a PACS system, use the worklist to select the patient.
4 Select the transducer:
   - abdomen/renal/transabdominal gynaecological scans: curvilinear broad-bandwidth probe with low central frequency (3–5 MHz)
   - transvaginal gynaecological scans: endovaginal broad-bandwidth probe with high central frequency (5–8 MHz)
   - testis/thyroid/vascular/breast/musculoskeletal scans: linear broad-bandwidth probe with high central frequency (6–17 MHz)
5 Select the application or 'preset' (the body part that is to be scanned). The machine then adjusts its postprocessing algorithm accordingly – e.g. 'carotid' will increase edge definition and contrast and decrease frame averaging.
6 Dim the ambient light levels in the room.
7 Apply an aqueous gel, which acts as a coupling medium, to the scan area.
8 Proceed to scan using the guidelines outlined in this book.
9 Optimize the image quality using the following functions:
   (a) Depth. Adjust this so the area of interest fills the screen.
   (b) Overall gain. Turning this up or down will adjust the overall image 'brightness'.
   (c) Focus. Place the focus position (indicated by a small marker on the side of the screen) to the bottom of the area of interest. By selecting two or three 'focal zones', the lateral resolution of the scan can be improved (e.g. good for testis, breast, musculoskeletal or TS kidney); however, the trade-off is a slower frame rate (slower image update).

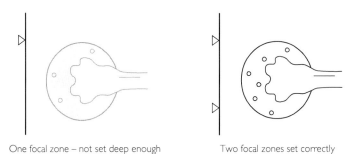

One focal zone – not set deep enough   Two focal zones set correctly

   (d) Time gain control (TGC). This amplifies weak returning echoes from varying depths and adjusts brightness at these levels. Start with the TGC in a vertical line in the middle of the scale and adjust from here – e.g., for bladder imaging, it can be adjusted to remove anterior wall reverberation artefacts: Most current machines have an automated program that adjusts the TGC in real time.

DOI: 10.1201/9781003381655-2

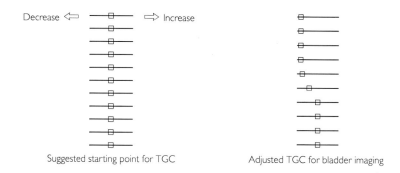

Suggested starting point for TGC   Adjusted TGC for bladder imaging

(e) Field of view (FOV). By reducing this to the smallest required area, the frame rate will be maximized, which increases the line density and thus improves image resolution:

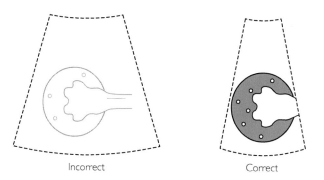

Incorrect   Correct

(f) Frequency. With a multifrequency transducer, the following options are available:
  (i) Increasing the frequency improves resolution of superficial structures
  (ii) Reducing the frequency improves penetration of deeper structures.

(g) Resolution/speed. This ranges from 1 to 5, and by setting it at 4 or 5, the detail in the image will be improved – but at the expense of a reduced frame rate,

(h) Tissue harmonics. This sharpens up images by reducing signal from the fat layers and improving edge definition but slows the frame rate, and may decrease the penetration.

(i) Compound imaging. This generally improves image quality by reducing artefact and improving boundary definition. However, it slows the frame rate.

(j) Zoom. This magnifies the screen image, which is useful for viewing small structures like ovaries. It can be used during dynamic scanning or when the image is frozen. It has no effect on the frame rate

(k) Parallel. This function is available on some machines. It improves resolution by sending out two signals side by side, which increases the frame rate and allows the use of multiple focal zones, which in turn improves the resolution.

(l) Acoustic (output) power. If overall gain and TGC are at maximum and it is still not possible to penetrate a structure (e.g. the liver), then try to increase this. However, the mechanical index (MI) and thermal index (TI) should always be kept to the lowest level which allows an image to be obtained.

(m) Doppler functions. These give blood flow information and can be used in several different ways:
  (i) *Colour Doppler.* A 'box' appears with a colour map of flow within vessels. Usually red and blue indicate flow towards and away from the probe respectively – but the operator can adjust this.
  (ii) *Power Doppler.* This is similar to colour Doppler but no directional information is given. It is more sensitive for detecting low-velocity flow.

(III) ***Spectral Doppler.*** When this is selected, a 'gate marker' appears, which the operator places over the vessel of interest to give detailed analysis of flow velocities at this site., A waveform above and below the baseline indicates flow towards and away from the probe respectively – the operator can reverse this if desired by selecting the 'spectral invert' function. The spectral Doppler trace can usually be displayed on screen alongside either a 'frozen' scan image or the 'real-time' image. The real-time image will have a slower frame rate than a regular colour image, but it can still be useful when trying to locate small vessels that are moving with respiration (e.g. renal interlobar arteries). In practice, most operators adjust between the two.

Optimizing colour Doppler

1 Select a probe that gives adequate penetration through to the region of interest. If flow cannot be seen, consider changing to a lower-frequency probe.
2 Ensure that the 'preset' (see above) is correct for the area being examined, as the machine adjusts the colour set-up and processing algorithm according to this.
3 Place the focus position at the level of the vessels of interest and reduce the size of the colour box to cover only this area.
4 If the colour signal is weak, try increasing the colour gain and reducing the colour box width and, on a curvilinear probe, the overall sector width.
5 Adjust the scale/pulse repetition frequency (PRF). This controls how frequently pulses are sent from the probe to detect flow:
    * for slow moving blood (e.g. venous), select low scale/PRF
    * for fast moving blood (e.g. arterial), select high scale/PRF
6 Adjust the filter settings to cut out signals below a certain frequency shift (this is good for removing noise). However, when trying to detect low flow velocities, the filter should be turned off/lowered – e.g. in cases of suspected testicular torsion.
7 Adjust the probe position until the angle between the beam and the vessel of interest is between 0° and 60° (see below).

Optimizing power Doppler. All of the above points apply, but as no velocity or directional flow is being measured, points 5 and 7 are not as important.

Optimizing spectral Doppler. The points listed above for colour Doppler are all important. In addition, to ensure accurate estimation of the flow velocity, ensure that the beam-flow angle is between 0° and 60°, because if the vessel is running at or near right angles, calculated velocities are unreliable (as cos 90° = 0).

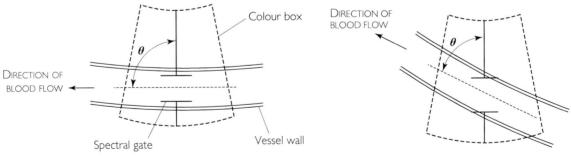

θ = 90°: incorrect angle between incident beam and direction of blood flow

θ<60°: improved angle between incident beam and direction of blood flow

Hint: When using a linear probe (e.g. veins or carotids), steer the colour box along the direction of flow in the vessel. Aim for a beam-flow angle <60° for accurate velocity calculations:

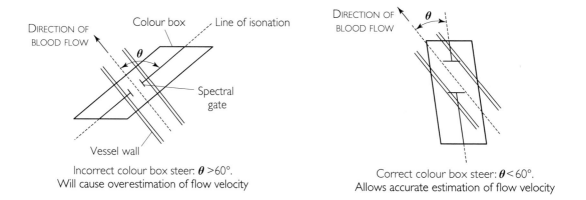

Incorrect colour box steer: $\theta > 60°$.
Will cause overestimation of flow velocity

Correct colour box steer: $\theta < 60°$.
Allows accurate estimation of flow velocity

2 The gate size (sample volume) should be adjusted to fill the whole vessel – e.g. if it is too big then signals from nearby vessels may be included:

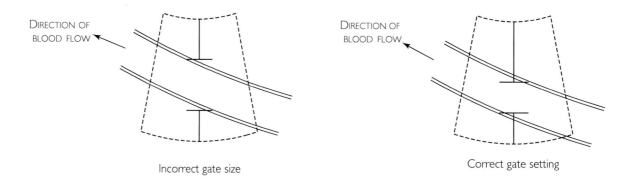

Incorrect gate size

Correct gate setting

(n) B-Flow, superb microvascular imaging. These are techniques for visualizing blood flow without using Doppler. They generally provide better sensitivity to low flow in small vessels than Doppler as there is an improved signal-to-noise ratio and there is a reduction in artefacts. They are emerging techniques and can be combined with the use of ultrasound contrast media.

(o) Contrast medium use. Microbubble agents resonate within the ultrasound beam and provide an increased amplitude of echo. There are special settings on machines to allow these to work. Notably, a low MI is needed to prevent destruction of the bubbles.

(p) M-mode function. When this is selected, a line appears, which the operator places across the site of interest. The display then shows only the echoes from this one line, but plotted against time. This reveals the movement of structures towards and away from the probe. It is used in early pregnancy scanning (see Chapter 11).

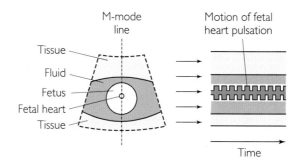

When the images appear to be satisfactory, start recording them:

10 Press the freeze button to get a still image.

11 Some systems allow review of the last few seconds before this via a 'ciné loop'.

12 Distances can be marked via the measurement function and tracker ball.

13 It is good practice to label images via either bodymarkers or typescript.

14 Once the examination is complete, end study on the machine and store/print images according to the set-up in the department – e.g. PACS, hardcopy, etc.

15 Ensure the transducer is thoroughly cleaned between patients using the appropriate cleaning solution/spray.

USEFUL ABDOMINAL ANATOMY

The complexity of the abdominal anatomy can be daunting, but it is not necessary to learn every relationship of each organ at once – start by learning the basics and then build up more detailed knowledge on this foundation. Here we summarize three TS sections at specific vertebral levels and three useful LS sections. Learn the important points from these schematic diagrams and then, through scanning experience, create a mental picture of the three-dimensional structure of the abdominal contents and their key relationships. Over time, as you acquire anatomical knowledge, you will begin to develop pattern recognition for what is normal and what is not.

TS: T12 vertebral level

Probe position:
immediately inferior to xiphisternum

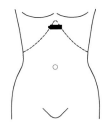

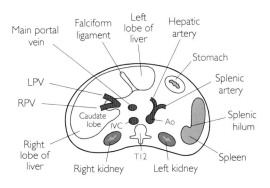

● *Key points*

1 The coeliac axis arises from the aorta at the T12 level.
2 The coeliac axis branches into the splenic artery and the hepatic artery – this branching appears as a 'seagull' shape when seen in TS.
3 The falciform ligament separates the liver into anatomical left and right lobes.
4 The splenic vein and superior mesenteric vein join to form the portal vein at T12/L1.
5 The portal vein branches into the right and left portal veins at the porta hepatis.

TS: L1 vertebral level

Probe position:
halfway between xiphisternum and umbilicus

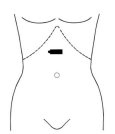

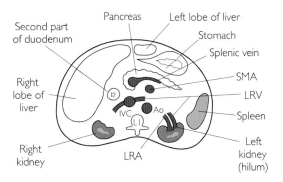

DOI: 10.1201/9781003381655-3

● *Key points*

1 The left renal hilum lies approximately 2 cm more superiorly than the right renal hilum.
2 The left renal vein passes anterior to the aorta.
3 The right renal artery passes posterior to the inferior vena cava.
4 The pancreas lies immediately anterior to the splenic vein.
5 The splenic vein is 'tadpole'-shaped when imaged in TS – i.e. the 'head' of the tadpole is the portal confluence and the 'tail' is the splenic vein.

TS: L2 vertebral level

Probe position:
just superior to the umbilicus

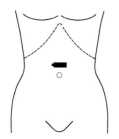

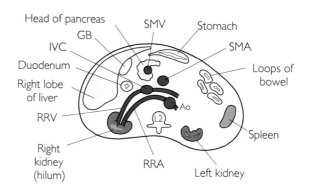

● *Key points*

1 The renal arteries branch off the aorta at L2.
2 The renal veins lie anterior to the renal arteries.
3 The superior mesenteric vein and splenic vein join to form the portal vein posterior to the neck of the pancreas.
4 The aorta bifurcates are just inferior to this level at L3/4.

LS: right MCL

Probe position:
midpoint of costal margin

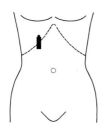

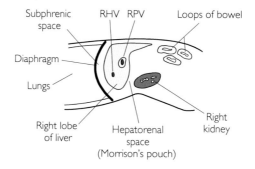

LS: right of midline

Probe position:
just right of midline over the costal margin

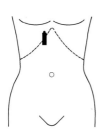

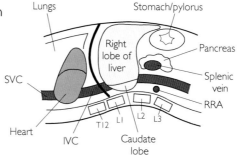

LS: left of midline

Probe position:
just left of midline over the costal margin

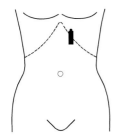

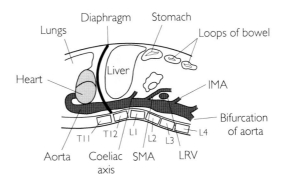

PERITONEAL SPACES

TS

Probe position:
L1 vertebral level, just below the xiphisternum

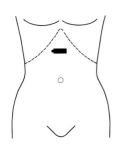

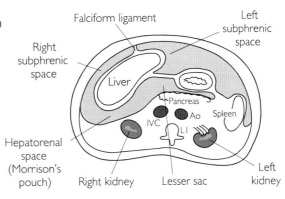

LS

Probe position:
just right of midline over the costal margin

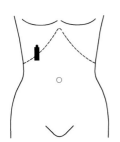

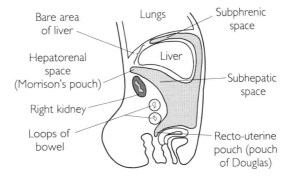

● Key points

1 The spaces are formed between folds of the peritoneum.
2 These spaces are where free fluid accumulates.
3 Morrison's pouch is the most dependent part of the abdominal cavity when the patient is supine. Therefore, ALWAYS examine here for free fluid.

ANATOMY OF THE PORTA HEPATIS AND BILIARY SYSTEM

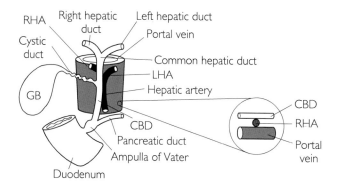

● *Key points*

1 The right hepatic artery runs between the common bile duct and portal vein in 90% of patients.
2 The right and left hepatic ducts join at the porta hepatis to form the common hepatic duct.
3 The common hepatic duct joins the cystic duct to form the common bile duct.
4 The common bile duct joins the pancreatic duct to form the ampulla of Vater, which empties into the duodenum.

ECHOGENICITY OF ABDOMINAL ORGANS

Remember the mnemonic PLiSK when comparing the echogenicity of the abdominal organs (see Chapter 1):

P Li S K

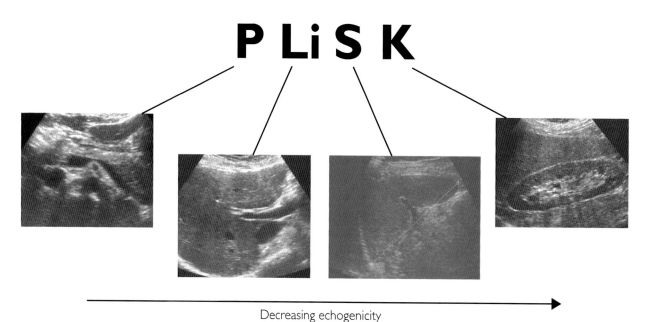

Decreasing echogenicity

SEGMENTS OF THE LIVER

Initially, it is acceptable to describe the position of abnormalities as either in the left or right lobe:

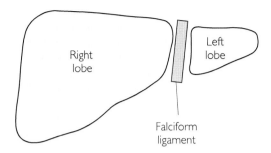

Eventually, however, it is worth learning the surgical segments of the liver in order to describe any abnormalities more accurately:

Viewed from above, the appearance is as follows:

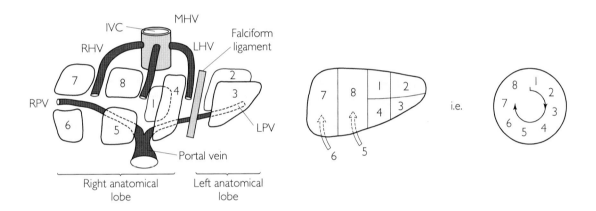

● Key points

1 The liver is divided into eight surgical segments by the branches of the portal and hepatic veins.
2 When viewed from above, the segments are numbered clockwise 1–8.
3 Segment 1 is the caudate lobe.
4 Segment 4 is a good place to look for focal fatty sparing or focal fatty infiltration.
5 Segment 6 extends beyond the inferior border of the right kidney in hepatomegaly.
6 75% of the liver's blood supply is from the portal vein and 25% from the hepatic artery.
7 The liver is drained via the three hepatic veins into the inferior vena cava.
8 Intrahepatic portal veins have echo-bright walls.

PERFORMING THE SCAN

- **Patient position**: Supine.
- **Preparation**: Nil by mouth or just clear fluids for 8 hours.
- **Probe**: Low-frequency (3–5 MHz) curvilinear.
- **Machine**: Select the abdomen preset mode. Use tissue harmonics and compound imaging if the SNR is poor or with obese patients.
- **Method**: Acquire more than just representative images for each step if pathology is found.

PROBE POSITION

INSTRUCTIONS

1 Midline – TS: pancreas

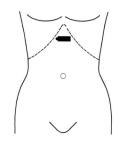

- Place the probe perpendicular to the upper abdomen in the midline. Look for the 'tadpole' shape of the splenic vein (tail) and portal confluence (head), and then look anterior to this to locate the pancreas.
- Scan through the whole pancreas by angling the probe cranially then caudally. Take note of the following pancreas characteristics:
  - size: is it swollen (acute pancreatitis)?
  - echogenicity (bright = fat infiltration)
  - any masses/cysts?
  - dilated pancreatic duct (>2 mm)?
  - any calcifications (chronic pancreatitis)?
- Acquire representative image(s).
- Pitfall: the 'dark' posterior muscular wall of the stomach can mimic the pancreatic duct.

2 Midline – LS: pancreas

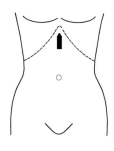

- Turn the probe 90° clockwise to scan in LS. Look for the splenic vein and then look anterior to this to locate the pancreas.
- Scan through the whole pancreas by angling the probe laterally right and left.
- If the pancreas cannot be found, try scanning:
  - again at the end of the examination
  - after filling the stomach with water
  - with the patient in the lateral decubitus position to move the overlying bowel out of the way
  - with the patient sitting erect
- Take note of the characteristics as listed in Step 1.
- Acquire representative image(s).

3 Midline – TS: aorta

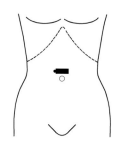

- Turn the probe 90° anticlockwise in order to scan in TS again.
- Increase the depth and look for the aorta.
- Turn on colour Doppler if there is difficulty in finding the aorta (especially in obese patients).
- Follow the course of the aorta down to the bifurcation, looking for any aneurysms or atherosclerosis.
- Measure the AP diameter of the aorta (inner wall to inner wall) at its widest point.
- Acquire representative image(s).

WHAT TO LOOK FOR

SCAN IMAGE

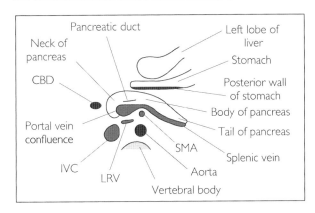

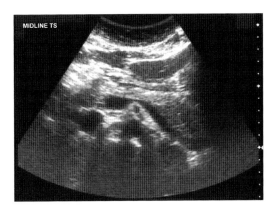

Tadpole head = portal vein confluence
Tadpole tail = splenic vein
Hint: Do not mistake the posterior wall of the stomach for a dilated pancreatic duct!

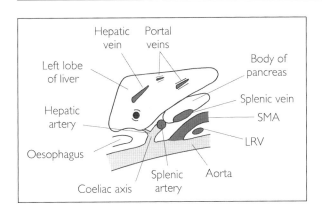

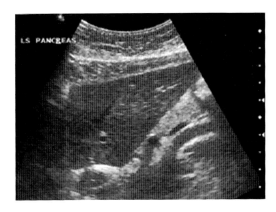

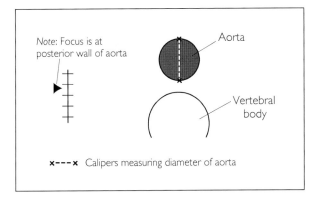

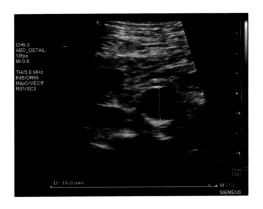

PROBE POSITION   **INSTRUCTIONS**

4 Midline – TS: left lobe of liver

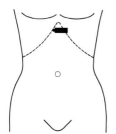

- Keep the probe TS and in the midline. Scan through the whole of the left lobe of the liver by angling the probe cranially and then caudally.
- Take note of:
  - the echogenicity: diffuse and focal
  - the size
  - the surface: is it smooth or nodular, is it cirrhotic?
  - the bile ducts: are they dilated?
  - any lesions: do they have mass effect?
  - hepatic and portal veins
- If there is difficulty in viewing the liver clearly, ask the patient to take a deep breath in to push the liver down.
- Acquire representative image(s).

5 LS: aorta and left lobe of liver

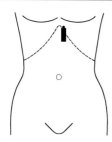

- Turn the probe 90° clockwise into LS and place it just left of the midline.
- Increase the depth as necessary and look for the aorta.
- Look for the SMA branching off and passing over the LRV.
- Examine the left lobe of the liver by sweeping the probe towards the LUQ.
- Make sure to scan completely off the liver edge, as this is a common place for metastases to 'hide'.
- Take note of the liver characteristics listed in Step 4.
- Acquire representative image(s).

6 LS: IVC and caudate

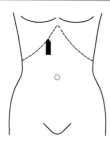

- Keep the probe in LS and move to the right of the midline.
- Look for the IVC passing through the liver with the caudate lobe anteriorly and posteriorly.
- Take note of the liver characteristics listed in Step 4.
- Examine the IVC for:
  - dilation with expiration (normal)
  - size (>2 cm AP diameter in CCF)
- Acquire representative image(s).

WHAT TO LOOK FOR

SCAN IMAGE

4

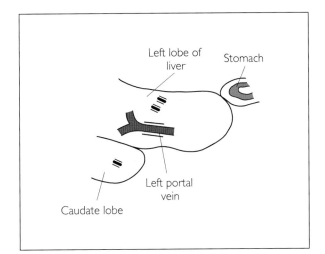

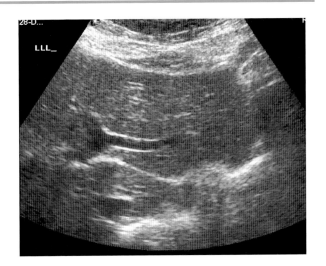

5

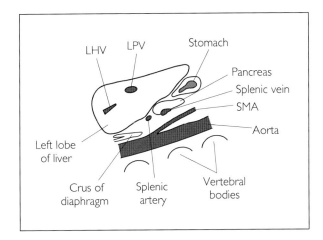

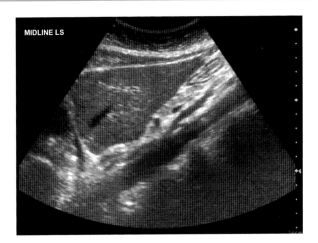

6

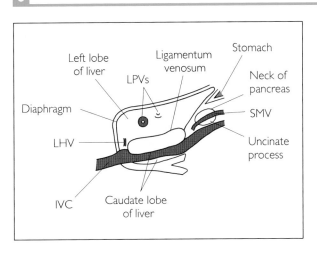

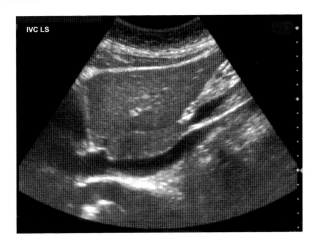

PROBE POSITION   **INSTRUCTIONS**

7 LS: porta hepatis and CBD measurement

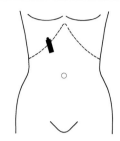

- Keep in LS and move the probe further to the patient's right.
- Take note of the liver characteristics listed in Step 4.
- Look for the portal vein and follow its course into the liver. The porta hepatis is the region where the vein enters the liver. At this point, look for the CBD by rotating the probe slightly anticlockwise and looking anterior to the portal vein. The hepatic artery runs between the duct and the portal vein (usually).
- To help locate the CBD:
  - turn on colour: no flow in CBD; remember to have a Doppler angle <60o
  - increase line density by reducing sector angle and depth
  - use zoom to magnify the area
- Follow the course of the CBD, looking for any calculi or obstruction.
- Measure the CBD at its widest point. It should be <6mm (or <9mm post-cholecystectomy).
- Look for lymph nodes at the porta hepatis.
- Acquire representative image(s).

8 LS: right liver medial to right kidney

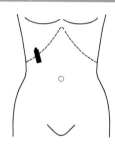

- Keep in LS and move the probe further to the patient's right. Sweep the probe laterally to the left and then right, examining the right lobe of the liver.
- Take note of the liver characteristics listed in Step 4.
- Look above and below the diaphragm for any pleural effusions/free fluid/subphrenic collections.
- Acquire representative image(s).

9 LS: right kidney/liver

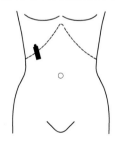

- Keep in LS and move the probe further to the right (usually MCL) to image the right kidney and the right lobe of the liver.
- Sweep laterally towards the RUQ, examining the liver characteristics. Make sure to scan completely off the right edge of the liver.
- Compare the echogenicity of the liver parenchyma and renal cortex (the liver should be a little brighter – remember PLiSK!).
- Look for hepatomegaly:
  - Does segment 6 of the liver extend below the inferior renal pole?
  - Is the angle of the liver >45°, i.e. rounded?
- Look for any fluid in the hepatorenal space (Morrison's pouch).
- Acquire representative image(s).

WHAT TO LOOK FOR   **SCAN IMAGE**

7

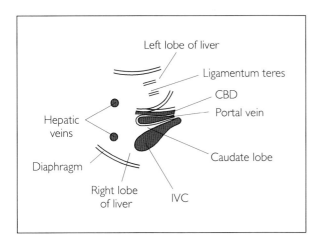

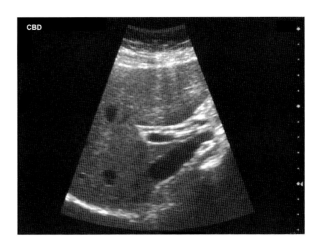

8

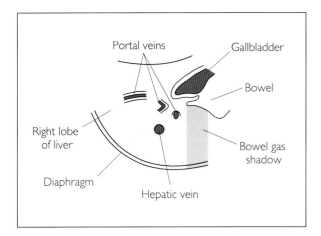

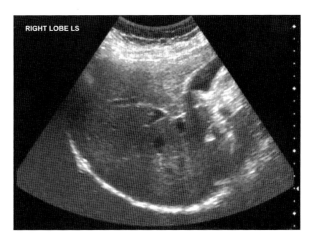

9

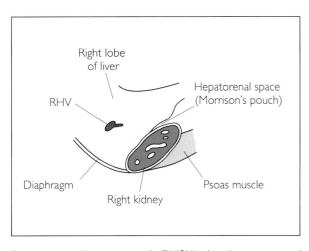

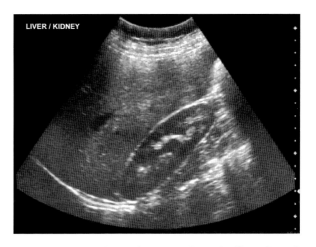

Remember the mnemonic PLiSK – i.e. the pancreas is normally the most echogenic organ, then the liver, then the spleen, then the kidney.

PROBE POSITION   **INSTRUCTIONS**

10 TS: liver – level of hepatic veins

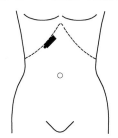

- Place the probe parallel and inferior to the right costal margin to scan the liver in TS.
- Ask the patient to take a deep breath in and at the same time angle the probe cranially under the costal margin to scan through the liver.
- Take note of the liver characteristics listed in Step 4.
- Look specifically for the hepatic veins and their confluence at the IVC. Take representative images of the right, middle and left hepatic veins.

11 TS: liver – level of porta hepatis

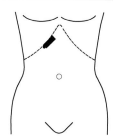

- Keep the probe parallel to the right costal margin.
- Ask the patient to take a deep breath in again. At the same time, angle the probe cranially under the costal margin, and sweep cranially then caudally to scan through the liver in TS.
- Take note of the liver characteristics listed in Step 4.
- Specifically examine the porta hepatis area for lymph nodes.
- Take representative image(s).

12 TS: liver – level of right kidney

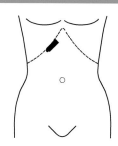

- Keep the probe parallel to the right costal margin.
- Ask the patient to take a deep breath in again. At the same time, angle the probe cranially under the costal margin, and sweep cranially then caudally to scan through the liver in TS.
- Take note of the liver characteristics listed in Step 4.
- Specifically examine the liver at the level of the right kidney.
- Make sure to scan inferiorly off the liver.
- Take representative image(s).

WHAT TO LOOK FOR

SCAN IMAGE

10

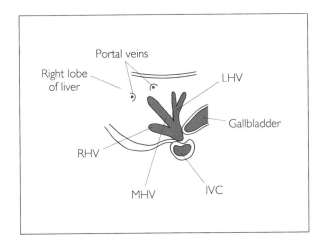

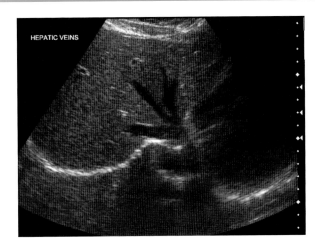

11

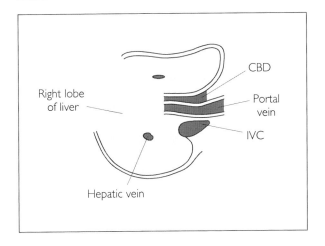

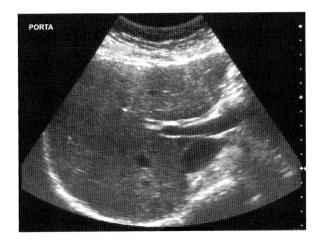

12

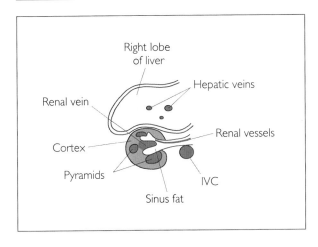

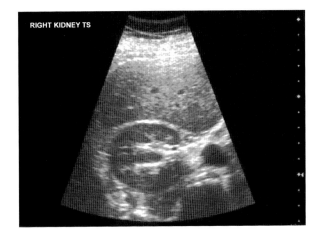

PROBE POSITION	**INSTRUCTIONS**

13 LS: gallbladder

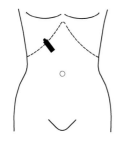

- Scan in the RUQ to find the GB – position varies in different patients.
- Rotate the probe so that the GB is imaged in its long axis.
- Now keep the probe face over the same area of skin, but angle the probe handle backwards and forwards to scan through the whole GB.
- Narrow the sector width and use multiple focal zones with or without zoom to improve detail.
- Take note of:
  - GB contents: calculi, sludge, polyps, gas, mass?
  - GB wall thickness (<3 mm?)
  - pericholecystic fluid
  - localized tenderness (Murphy's sign)
- If something can be seen within the GB, move the patient and rescan to see if it has moved with gravity (calculi/sludge vs polyp/mass). It is vital in any case to examine the gallbladder with the patient in more than one position to ensure any 'hidden' gallstones fall into view.
- Measure any abnormalities seen.
- Acquire representative images.

14 TS: gallbladder

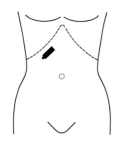

- Scan the GB in TS: to do this, first scan it in LS and then rotate the probe anticlockwise through 90° to image in TS.
- Now keep the probe face over the same area of skin, but angle the probe handle backwards and forwards to scan through the whole GB in TS.
- Narrow the sector width and use multiple focal zones with or without zoom to improve detail.
- Take note of the GB characteristics listed in Step 13.
- If something can be seen within the GB, try moving the patient and rescanning to see if it has moved with gravity (calculi/sludge vs polyp/mass).
- Measure any abnormalities seen.
- Acquire at least three representative images.

WHAT TO LOOK FOR   **SCAN IMAGE**

13

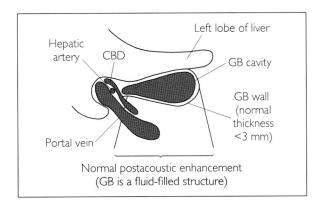

Hepatic artery
CBD
Left lobe of liver
GB cavity
GB wall (normal thickness <3 mm)
Portal vein
Normal postacoustic enhancement (GB is a fluid-filled structure)

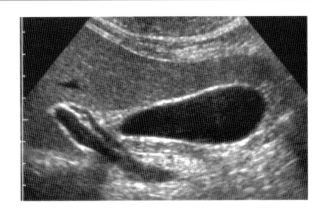

14

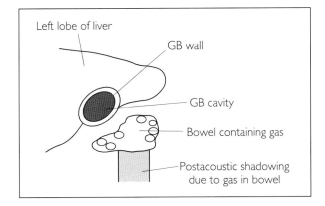

Left lobe of liver
GB wall
GB cavity
Bowel containing gas
Postacoustic shadowing due to gas in bowel

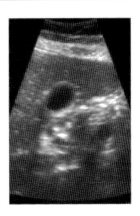

PROBE POSITION   **INSTRUCTIONS**

15 LS: right kidney

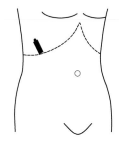

- Turn the patient 45° onto their left side.
- Place the probe in the RUQ and ask the patient to breathe in and hold.
- Locate the right kidney in LS. If there is difficulty finding it, try a more posterolateral approach. If rib shadows interfere, try scanning with the probe angled along a rib space.
- Scan through the kidney in LS, observing:
  - cortical thickness and echogenicity
  - medullary pyramids
  - pelvicalyceal system
- Are there any masses, cysts, calculi or hydronephrosis?
- Measure any abnormalities seen.
- Measure the greatest kidney length (pole-to-pole).
- Acquire at least two representative images.

16 TS: right kidney

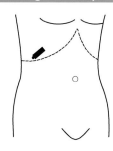

- Turn the probe 90° anticlockwise to scan in TS.
- Narrow the FOV and use two focal zones, with the second at the posterior aspect of the kidney.
- Ask the patient to breathe in and hold.
- Scan through the right kidney in TS and take note of the kidney characteristics listed in Step 15.
- If bowel gas shadows interfere, ask the patient to push out the abdomen or press over the kidney with your free hand to displace the bowel.
- Measure any abnormalities seen.
- Acquire at least two representative images.

17 LS: spleen

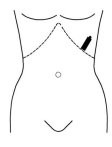

- Ask the patient to lie either 45° on the right side or supine. It is best to scan the spleen with the patient gently breathing. To find the spleen, place the probe in the 9th ICS AAL.
- Sweep the probe posteriorly and anteriorly to scan through the whole spleen in LS.
- Take note of:
  - echogenicity compared with the left kidney (the spleen should be brighter)
  - texture (fine homogenous = normal)
  - any masses/infarcts/varices
- Measure the spleen size from tip to tip.
- Acquire representative image(s).

WHAT TO LOOK FOR   **SCAN IMAGE**

15

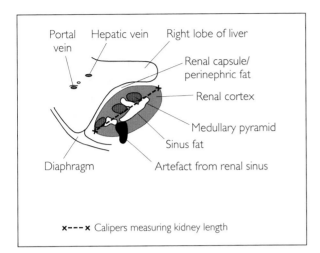

- Portal vein
- Hepatic vein
- Right lobe of liver
- Renal capsule/perinephric fat
- Renal cortex
- Medullary pyramid
- Sinus fat
- Diaphragm
- Artefact from renal sinus

×---× Calipers measuring kidney length

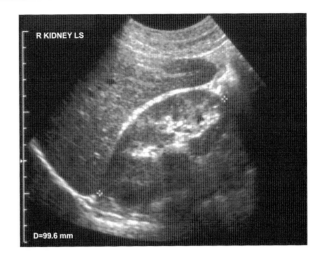

16

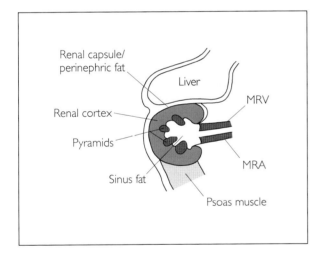

- Renal capsule/perinephric fat
- Liver
- MRV
- Renal cortex
- Pyramids
- MRA
- Sinus fat
- Psoas muscle

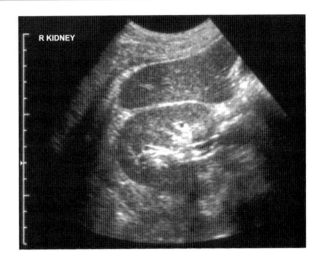

17

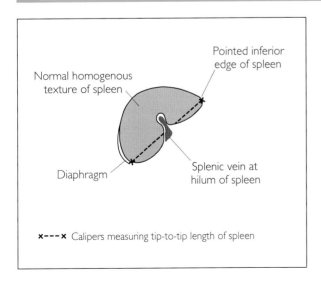

- Normal homogenous texture of spleen
- Pointed inferior edge of spleen
- Splenic vein at hilum of spleen
- Diaphragm

×---× Calipers measuring tip-to-tip length of spleen

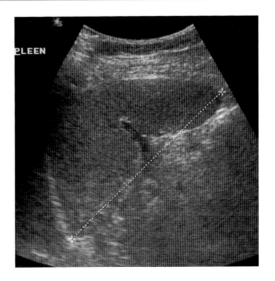

PROBE POSITION	**INSTRUCTIONS**

18 TS: spleen

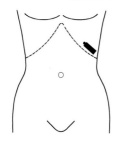

- Find the spleen in LS and then rotate the probe through 90° anticlockwise to image it in TS.
- Sweep the probe superiorly and inferiorly to scan through the whole spleen, ensuring the diaphragmatic surface is seen in its entirety.
- Take note of the spleen characteristics listed in Step 17.
- Measure any abnormalities seen.
- Acquire representative image(s).
- Occasionally, the left lobe of the liver can extend across and lie between the spleen and diaphragm. Take care not to mistake this for a mass/lesion.

19 LS: left kidney

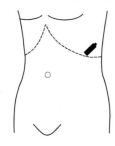

- Turn the patient 45° onto the right side.
- Place the probe obliquely over the LUQ and ask the patient to breathe in and hold.
- Look for the left kidney in LS with the spleen adjacent to it for comparison of echogenicity (the spleen should be brighter).
- *Hint:* The left kidney is higher and more posterior than the right – the 11th ICS is a good landmark.
- Scan through the left kidney in LS, observing:
  - cortical thickness and echogenicity
  - medullary pyramids
  - pelvicalyceal system
- Are there any masses, cysts, calculi or hydronephrosis?
- Measure any abnormalities seen.
- Measure the greatest kidney length (pole-to-pole).
- Acquire at least two representative images.

20 TS: left kidney

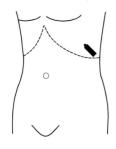

- Turn the probe 90° anticlockwise to scan in TS.
- Narrow the FOV and use two focal zones with the second at the posterior aspect of the kidney.
- Ask the patient to breathe in and hold.
- Scan through the left kidney in TS and take note of the kidney characteristics listed in Step 19.
- If bowel gas shadows interfere, ask the patient to push their abdomen out or press over the kidney with your free hand to displace the bowel.
- Measure any abnormalities seen.
- Acquire at least two representative images.

WHAT TO LOOK FOR

SCAN IMAGE

18

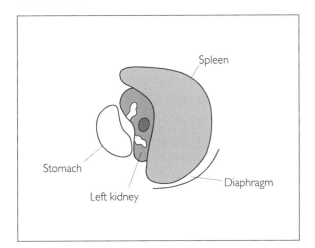

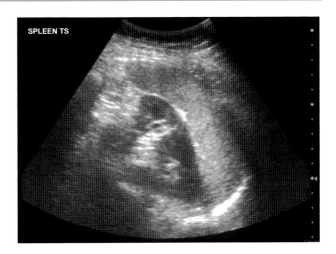

19

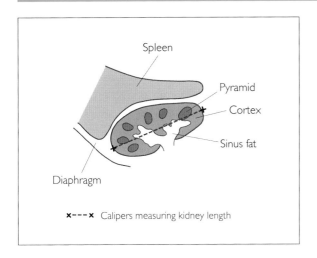

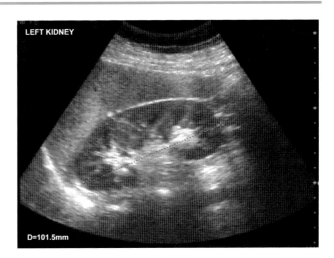

20

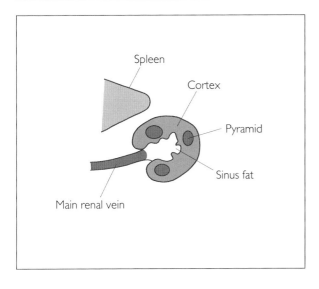

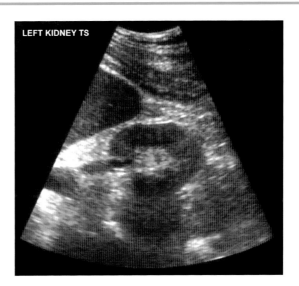

WHAT TO LOOK FOR

SCAN IMAGE

ABDOMEN PROTOCOLS

Below is a summary of the abdomen protocols described in this chapter – Protocol A. This is just one of many different protocols that can be used and other suggested abdomen protocols are summarized, with a list of advantages and disadvantages for each one. They differ in the sequence but all encompass a whole examination of the abdomen in at least two planes. Remember to move or turn the patient as appropriate for each view. We recommend that an operator picks one of the protocols, learns it and sticks to it – that way nothing will be missed out. It does not really matter which protocol is used, as long as you are methodical, consistent and thorough.

Abdomen protocol A

Midline	1	TS: pancreas
	2	LS: pancreas
	3	TS: aorta
	4	TS: left lobe of liver
LS: sweep across RUQ	5	LS: aorta and left lobe of the liver
	6	LS: IVC and caudate
	7	LS: porta hepatis and CBD
	8	LS: right liver medial to right kidney
	9	LS: right kidney/liver
TS: liver	10	Level of hepatic veins
	11	Level of porta hepatis
	12	Level of right kidney
Gallbladder	13	LS
	14	TS
Right kidney	15	LS
	16	TS
Spleen	17	LS
	18	TS
Left kidney	19	LS
	20	TS

Abdomen protocol B

LS sweep across RUQ	1	Liver/right kidney
	2	Liver medial to right kidney
	3	Porta hepatis
	4	CBD (and measurement)
	5	IVC and caudate
	6	Aorta and left lobe of liver
Midline	7	LS: left lobe of liver
	8	LS: pancreas
	9	LS: aorta
	10	TS: pancreas
	11	TS: aorta
TS liver	12	Left lobe of liver
	13	Level of hepatic veins/IVC
	14	Level of porta hepatis
	15	Level of right kidney
Gallbladder	16	LS
	17	TS
Right kidney	18	LS
	19	TS
Spleen	20	LS
	21	TS
Left kidney	22	LS
	23	TS

Abdomen protocol C

Pancreas	1	TS		10	Right lobe at level of porta hepatis
	2	LS			
Liver LS	3	LS: left lobe of liver		11	Left lobe of liver
	4	LS: IVC and caudate	Gallbladder	12	LS
	5	LS: porta hepatis and CBD		13	TS
	6	LS: right lobe of liver	Spleen	14	LS
Right kidney	7	LS		15	TS
	8	TS	Left kidney	16	LS
Liver TS	9	Right lobe at level of hepatic veins		17	TS
			Aorta	18	TS

EVALUATION OF ABDOMEN PROTOCOLS

Protocol	Advantages	Disadvantages
A	• There is an improved chance of visualizing the midline structures • Visualizing the pancreas is a confidence booster • Small amounts of ascites will have had time to accumulate in the hepatorenal space	• It is not possible to set up the system to assess liver echotexture – especially in patients with a 'fatty liver', when the left lobe may be echo-bright. In this case, the overall gain may be reduced to assess this lobe. Then, when the right lobe is assessed, the overall gain must be increased. As a result, it may not be possible to determine which lobe is abnormal
B	• The size of the liver is known immediately • A plan of the scan – all-intercostal for the right lobe or a combination of sub-/intercostal – can be made • An immediate note of moderate/large amount of ascites can be made	• Repeat inspiration and breathhold techniques may lead to midline structures being obscured by bowel gas • Small amounts of ascites may not have accumulated in the dependent hepatorenal space
C	• There is an improved chance of visualizing the pancreas (a confidence booster) • Viewing all right-sided structures in LS first and then in TS is simple to remember • Fewer probe rotations are needed, which can speed up scan time • Small amounts of ascites will have had time to accumulate in the hepatorenal space	• It is less sensitive for subtle abnormalities of liver echotexture • Liver scanning is interrupted to look at the right kidney. With this discontinuity, it is important to review any suspicious areas seen in the LS liver images

LIVER: PATHOLOGY

● 1 *Hepatomegaly*

Common causes are malignancy, infection and right heart failure.

Ultrasound features
- Segment 6 of the liver extends below the inferior pole of the right kidney (in LS)
- Segment 6 has a rounded margin (i.e. angle >45°)
- Both right and left lobes tend to be enlarged

Hint: Do not confuse hepatomegaly with Riedel's lobe (a congenitally large segment 6).

Ultrasound features of Riedel's lobe
- Segment 6 of the liver extends beyond the inferior pole of the right kidney (in LS)
- Segment 6 has a pointed margin (i.e. angle < 45°)
- The left lobe of the liver tends to be small

● 2 *Fatty liver (hepatic steatosis)*

Fatty infiltration of the liver is a very common finding. Causes include obesity, alcoholism and diabetes. It can be diffuse or focal. If focal, it is usually found in segment 4, adjacent to the porta.

Ultrasound features
- Bigger liver
- Brighter liver (i.e. much brighter than renal cortex)
- Loss of portal vein wall definition
- Post-attenuation fallout

WHAT TO LOOK FOR

SCAN IMAGE

1a Hepatomegaly

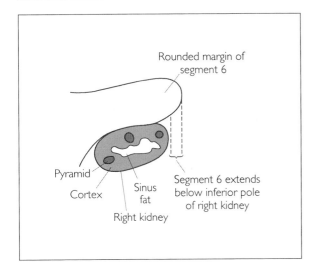

Rounded margin of
segment 6

Pyramid

Cortex

Sinus
fat

Right kidney

Segment 6 extends
below inferior pole
of right kidney

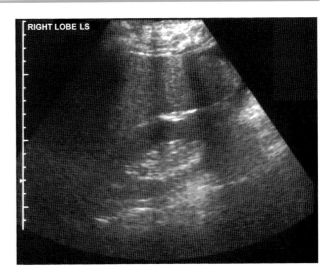

RIGHT LOBE LS

1b Riedel's lobe

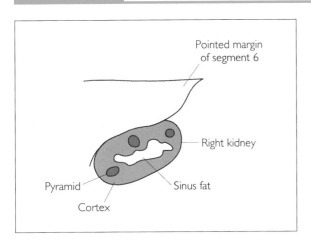

Pointed margin
of segment 6

Right kidney

Pyramid

Sinus fat

Cortex

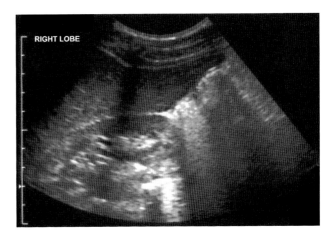

RIGHT LOBE

2 Fatty liver

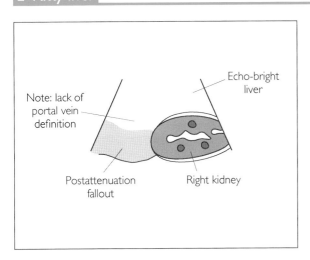

Note: lack of
portal vein
definition

Echo-bright
liver

Postattenuation
fallout

Right kidney

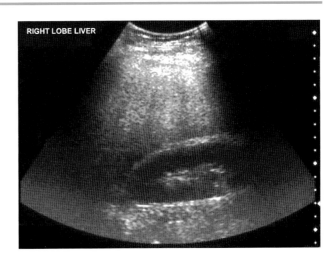

RIGHT LOBE LIVER

● 3 Focal fat sparing

Just as a normal liver can have focal fatty infiltration, sometimes a diffusely fat liver can have focal sparing.

Ultrasound features
- Usually affects segments 1 or 4
- Is seen as a relatively echo-poor area
- Has an irregular edge
- Has no mass effect
- May mimic a cyst

● 4 Metastases

Liver metastases are commonly from a primary malignancy of colon, stomach, breast or lung.

Ultrasound features
- Wide variation in appearance
- May be single or multiple, cystic or solid
- Echo-poor, echo-bright or a mass of mixed echogenicity
- Gastrointestinal primary tumours commonly give echo-bright metastases. These can have a 'target' appearance due to an echo-poor rim of oedema.
- Exhibit mass effect with disruption of normal anatomy
- Occasionally show neovascularization (tortuous new vessels seen with colour Doppler)

WHAT TO LOOK FOR

SCAN IMAGE

3 Focal fatty sparing

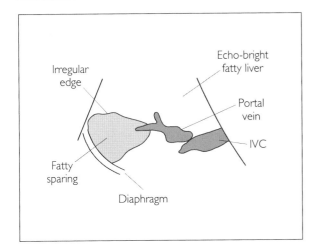

- Irregular edge
- Echo-bright fatty liver
- Portal vein
- IVC
- Fatty sparing
- Diaphragm

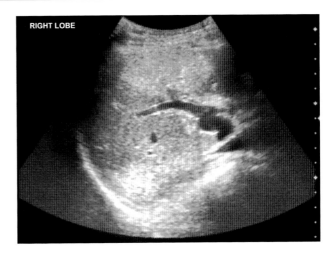

RIGHT LOBE

4a Liver metastases

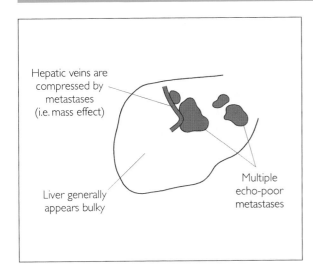

- Hepatic veins are compressed by metastases (i.e. mass effect)
- Liver generally appears bulky
- Multiple echo-poor metastases

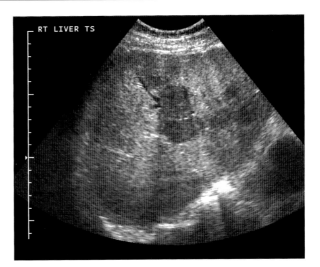

RT LIVER TS

4b Liver metastases

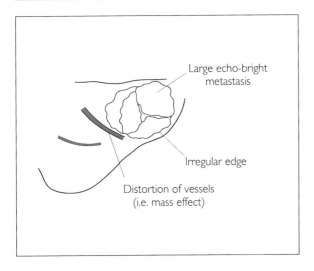

- Large echo-bright metastasis
- Irregular edge
- Distortion of vessels (i.e. mass effect)

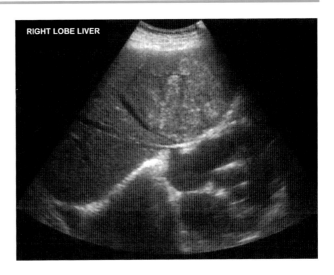

RIGHT LOBE LIVER

● 5 Cirrhosis

This is chronic liver disease resulting in fibrosis of liver parenchyma and nodule formation. Alcohol is the most common cause followed by chronic hepatitis B and C infection.

Ultrasound features
- Small contracted liver
- Irregular and nodular surface
- Increased parenchymal echotexture, which can be:
  - coarse, i.e. micronodular cirrhosis
  - contain discrete echo-poor nodules > 1 cm: i.e. macronodular cirrhosis
- Also look carefully for:
  - evidence of portal hypertension: ascites; splenomegaly; varices
  - associated hepatocellular carcinoma

WHAT TO LOOK FOR

SCAN IMAGE

5a Early cirrhosis

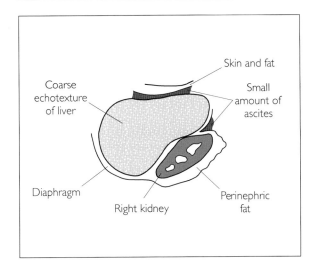

Coarse echotexture of liver

Skin and fat

Small amount of ascites

Diaphragm

Right kidney

Perinephric fat

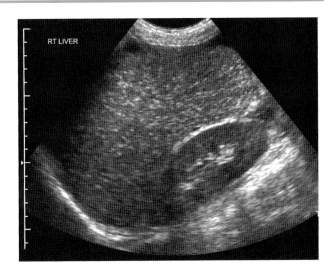

RT LIVER

5b End-stage cirrhosis

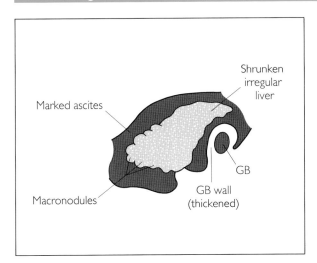

Marked ascites

Shrunken irregular liver

GB

GB wall (thickened)

Macronodules

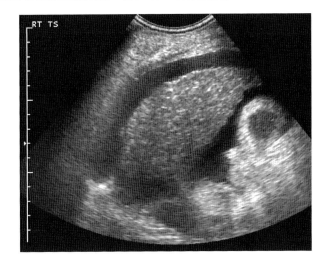

RT TS

● 6 Hepatocellular carcinoma

This is the most common primary liver cancer. The majority of HCCs occur in cirrhotic livers (see Page 32) which can make their detection very difficult due to the background changes.

Ultrasound features

- Usually in a cirrhotic liver
- Small HCCs are echo-poor
- Larger HCCs are echo-bright due to internal haemorrhage and necrosis
- Diffuse HCCs cause a generalized echotexture abnormality and can be easily missed
- Look for indirect evidence of tumour e.g. localized surface bulge

Hint: Always look for tumour thrombus within the portal and hepatic veins, and check for the patency of flow within these vessels (60% invade the PV; 25% invade HVs).

● 7 Hepatic cysts

These can be congenital or acquired. They are of no clinical significance unless associated with PCKD.

Ultrasound features

- Smooth edge
- Thin wall
- Echo-free contents
- Postacoustic enhancement

WHAT TO LOOK FOR　　　　　　　　**SCAN IMAGE**

6 Multiple HCCs

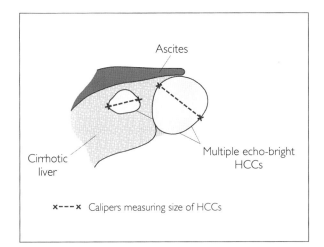

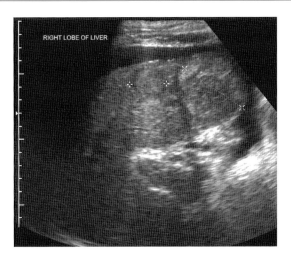

7 Simple hepatic cyst

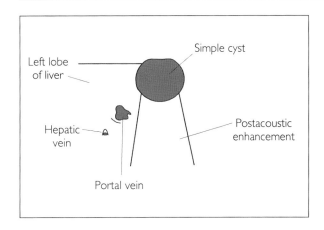

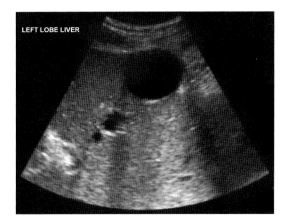

● 8 Liver abscess

This is a localized collection of pus within the liver. The majority are pyogenic and secondary to ascending infection, e.g. cholangitis, diverticulitis, etc. They can also result from bloodborne sepsis such as endocarditis. Rarely are they caused by amoebic or hydatid disease.

Ultrasound features
- Irregular outline due to debris and 'sick' liver. There is no true wall.
- Echo-poor lesion
- Contain 'lumpy' echo-bright debris
- Display variable postacoustic enhancement
- If the abscess contains gas intense reverberations are seen

● 9 Haemangioma

These are benign vascular lesions comprising multiple tiny blood vessels. They are a common incidental finding (5% of population). 80% occur in females.

Ultrasound features
- Usually small (<4 cm) well-defined echo-bright lesions
- Can appear echo-poor
- Postacoustic enhancement is common
- Slowly flowing blood – therefore appear avascular with colour/power Doppler

● 10 Congestive hepatopathy (or right heart failure alone)

This is hepatic congestion secondary to elevated right heart pressures. Causes include COPD, left ventricular failure and constrictive pericarditis.

Ultrasound features
- Dilated hepatic veins
- Dilated IVC (>2 cm AP diameter)
- Loss of IVC movement with respiration

WHAT TO LOOK FOR

SCAN IMAGE

8 Liver abscess

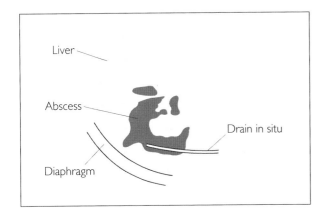

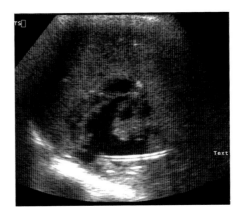

9 Haemangioma

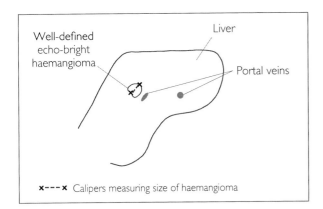

x---x Calipers measuring size of haemangioma

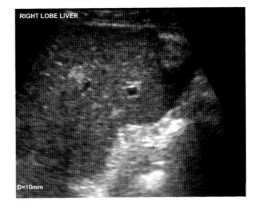

10 Congestive hepatopathy

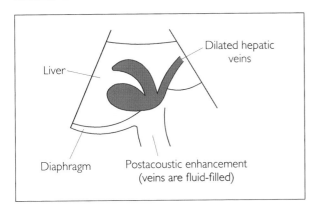

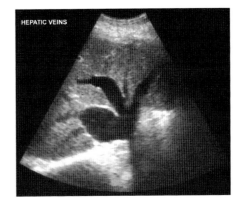

GALLBLADDER AND BILIARY TREE: PATHOLOGY

● 1 Gallstones

Cholesterol stones
- Risk factors: 'female, fat, over forty'
- Characteristics: large solitary stone

Pigmented stones
- Risk factors: haemolysis (considered in patients with sickle cell disease)
- Characteristics: small, irregular and multiple

Ultrasound features
- Echo-bright
- Well-defined
- Postacoustic shadowing
- Move to most dependent part with change in patient's position (cf. polyps)

How to distinguish a collapsed gallbladder around stones vs air in the bowel?
- Echoes from duodenal wall can resemble the gallbladder wall and air in the lumen causes distal shadowing
- Wall echo sign is specific for gallstones: this describes 2 parallel curvilinear lines (near line = gallbladder wall; far line = gallstone) separated by a thin echo-poor space (bile) with postacoustic shadowing
- Peristalsis is specific for the bowel

● 2 Cholecystitis

This is an infection of the gallbladder. 95% of cases have gallstones; 5% have sludge; acalculous cholecystitis (in ICU patients) is rare.

Ultrasound features
- Tender gallbladder
- Murphy's sign positive – patient catches breath on deep inspiration as gallbladder descends pushing against the probe
- Presence of stones or sludge (>95% of cases)
- Gallbladder wall thickness >3 mm
- Oedematous wall with indistinct outline
- Rim of echo-free pericholecystic fluid (also look in Morrison's pouch for free fluid)

Causes of gallbladder wall thickening
- Cholecystitis
- Ascites
- Hepatitis
- AIDS, postprandial, adenomyomatosis, tumour, leukaemic infiltration, hypoproteinaemia, Crohn's, Schistosomiasis, etc.

WHAT TO LOOK FOR   SCAN IMAGE

1a Gallstone

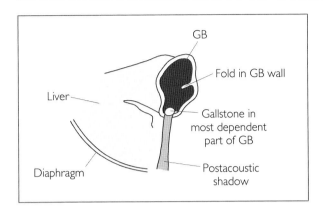

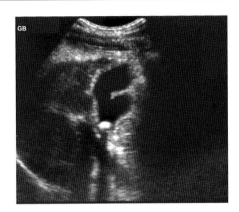

1b Biliary sludge

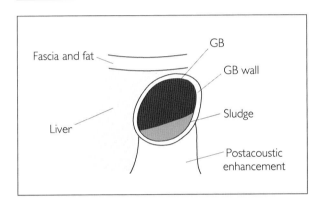

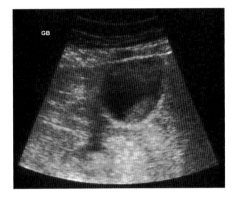

2 Cholecystitis

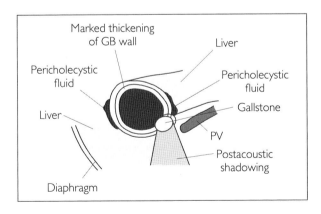

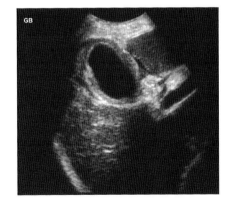

● *3 Biliary obstruction*

Most common causes
- Intrinsic: gallstones, cholangiocarcinoma, stricture, sclerosing cholangitis
- Extrinsic: acute pancreatitis, lymph nodes, carcinoma of the head of the pancreas

Ultrasound features
- 'Double-barrelled shotgun' sign of dilated bile duct radicals parallel to PV branches in the liver
- Dilation of ducts proximal to the obstruction
- If obstruction is distal the CBD will also be dilated (>6 mm or >9 mm postcholecystectomy)
- Ampullary obstruction (e.g. pancreatic carcinoma) causes 'double duct' sign of dilated CBD and dilated pancreatic duct (>2 mm)
- Look carefully for cause of obstruction e.g. gallstones, tumour

Hint: Scanning in the left lateral position and using the gallbladder as a window can help improve visualization of the distal CBD.

● *4 Gallbladder polyps*

These occur in 5% of the population and are usually asymptomatic. They are usually benign, but need monitoring as there is a risk of carcinoma developing in larger polyps.

Ultrasound features
- Echo-bright and well-defined
- No postacoustic shadowing
- Sometimes on a stalk
- Do not move to the most dependent part of the gallbladder (cf. gallstones)

Hint: Sit the patient up and rescan to see if the polyp/stone etc. has moved.

Hint: A polyp larger than 8 mm is considered pre-malignant and warrants surgical referral.

WHAT TO LOOK FOR   **SCAN IMAGE**

3a Biliary obstruction: stone in CBD

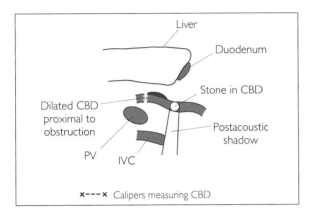

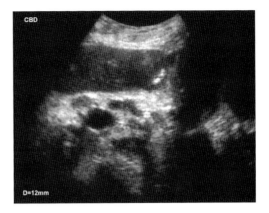

3b Biliary obstruction: dilated CBD

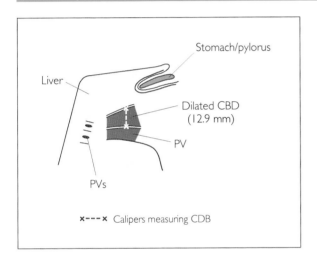

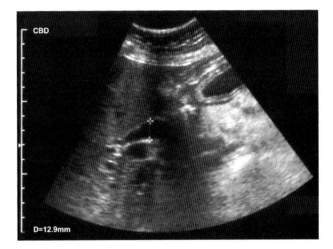

4 Gallbladder polyps

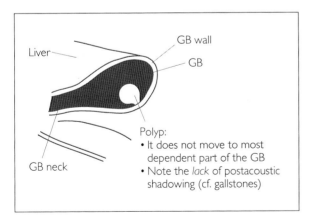

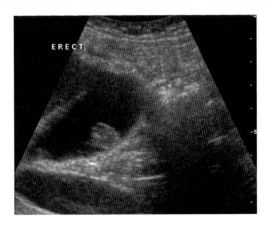

● 5 Adenomyomatosis

This benign condition is associated with gallstones. There is hyperplasia of the gallbladder wall epithelium resulting in mucosal diverticulae that extend into the muscular layer. The diverticulae are seen within the wall as fluid- or crystal-filled spaces.

Ultrasound features
- GB wall thickening can be diffuse or focal
- Diverticulae containing bile are echo-poor
- Diverticulae containing stones/sludge give a 'comet tail' artefact

● 6 Cholecystic carcinoma

This uncommon gastrointestinal malignancy has an increased prevalence in women and the elderly.

Ultrasound features
- Often associated with gallstones
- Gallbladder wall thickening in early disease
- GB is replaced by a mass of mixed echogenicity in later disease

● 7 Pneumobilia

This is air in the biliary tree. The commonest causes are iatrogenic (surgery, ERCP, etc.), cholecystenteric fistula and gallstone ileus.

Ultrasound features
- Reflective linear echoes within the biliary tree
- Ill-defined reverberation shadows seen posterior to the air

WHAT TO LOOK FOR　　　　　　　　**SCAN IMAGE**

5 Adenomyomatosis

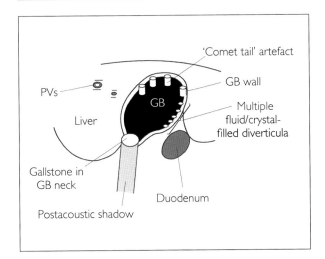

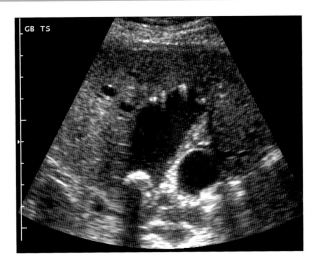

6 Cholecystic carcinoma

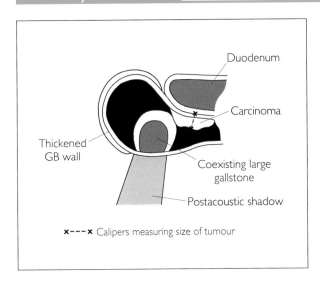

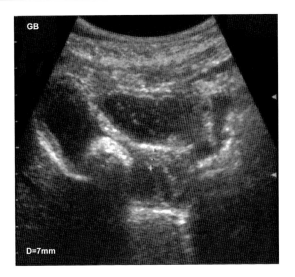

7 Pneumobilia

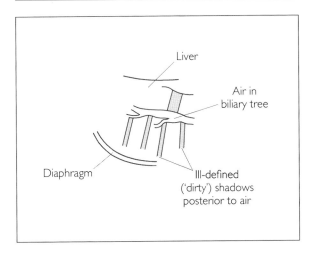

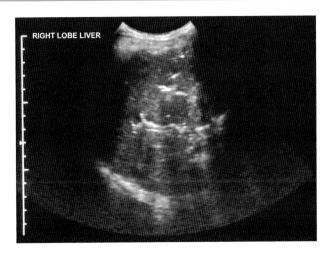

PANCREAS: PATHOLOGY

● 1 Acute pancreatitis

The most common causes are alcohol, gallstones, steroids, autoimmune causes and trauma.

Ultrasound features
- Swollen/enlarged pancreas
- Echo-poor and difficult to visualize
- Tender over midline
- Fluid in flanks

Hint: Look carefully for a stone in the ampulla of Vater as these patients will be candidates for ERCP-guided stone removal.

● 2 Chronic pancreatitis

The most common cause is chronic alcohol abuse. Rarer causes include cystic fibrosis and autoimmune disease.

Ultrasound features
- Small atrophic echo-bright pancreas
- Speckled calcification
- Dilated pancreatic duct (60% cases)

Three causes of an echo-bright pancreas
- Advanced age
- Cystic fibrosis
- Chronic pancreatitis

● 3 Pancreatic carcinoma

This occurs usually in patients >40 years old and typically presenting with pain radiating through to the back, with or without jaundice. 65% of carcinomas are found in the head of the pancreas (>body>tail).

Ultrasound features
- Irregular mass
- Usually echo-poor
- Disruption of normal anatomy
- Double-duct sign (i.e. dilated CBD and pancreatic duct)

WHAT TO LOOK FOR

SCAN IMAGE

1 Acute pancreatitis

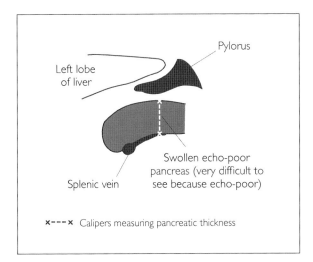

- Pylorus
- Left lobe of liver
- Swollen echo-poor pancreas (very difficult to see because echo-poor)
- Splenic vein

x---x Calipers measuring pancreatic thickness

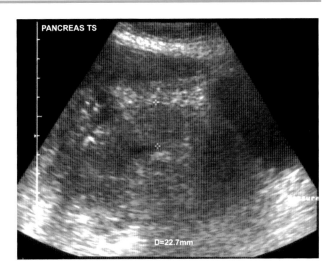

PANCREAS TS

D=22.7mm

2 Chronic pancreatitis

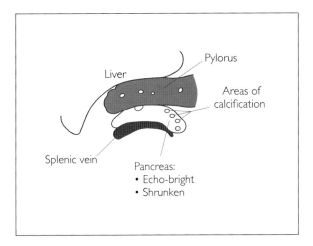

- Pylorus
- Liver
- Areas of calcification
- Splenic vein
- Pancreas:
  • Echo-bright
  • Shrunken

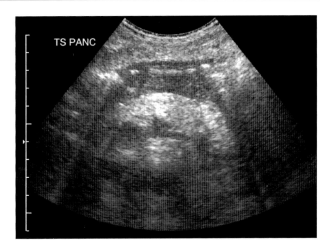

TS PANC

3 Pancreatic carcinoma

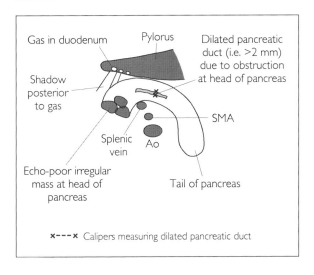

- Gas in duodenum
- Pylorus
- Dilated pancreatic duct (i.e. >2 mm) due to obstruction at head of pancreas
- Shadow posterior to gas
- SMA
- Splenic vein
- Ao
- Echo-poor irregular mass at head of pancreas
- Tail of pancreas

x---x Calipers measuring dilated pancreatic duct

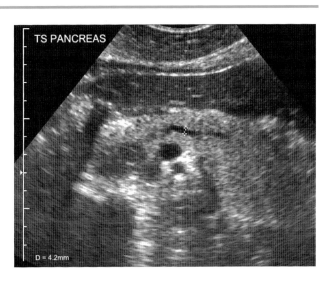

TS PANCREAS

D = 4.2mm

SPLEEN: PATHOLOGY

● *1 Splenunculus*

This is accessory spleen tissue. It occurs in 10% of the population and is an incidental finding of no clinical significance.

Ultrasound features
- Spherical
- Well-defined smooth outline
- Same echogenicity and echotexture as spleen
- Usually found at hilum

● *2 Splenomegaly*

The most common causes in the UK are portal hypertension, malignancy (lymphoma, leukaemia and myelofibrosis) and infection.

Ultrasound features
- >13 cm when measured from inferior pole tip to superior pole tip
- Inferior margin becomes rounded
- Look for clues as to the cause e.g. ascites, cirrhosis, lymph nodes

Hint: Asking the patient to place their left arm behind their head widens the intercostal space, hence opening up the scan window and making it easier to assess the spleen.

● *3 Lymphoma*

This is the most common malignancy of the spleen.

Ultrasound features
- Splenomegaly
- Associated lymphadenopathy in the abdomen
- Solitary or multiple echo-poor lesions in the splenic parenchyma

WHAT TO LOOK FOR

SCAN IMAGE

1 Splenunculus

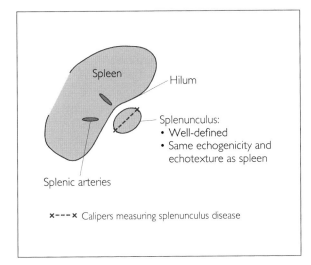

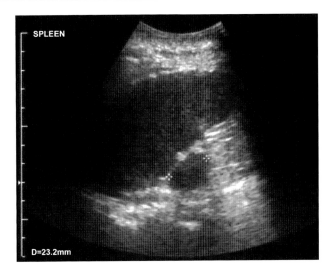

2 Splenomegaly

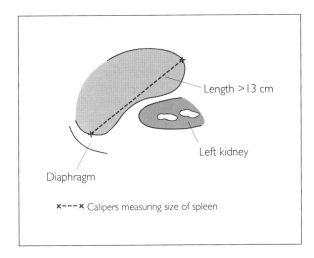

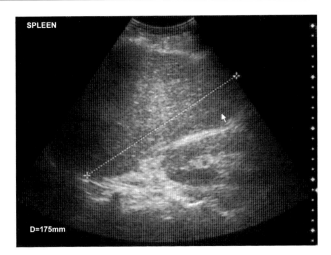

3 Lymphoma

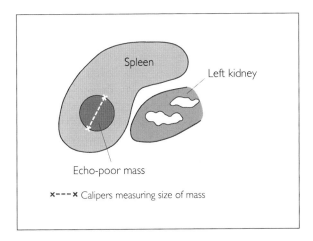

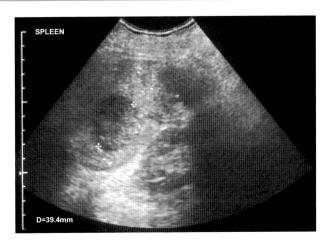

4 Renal and renal transplant

ANATOMY

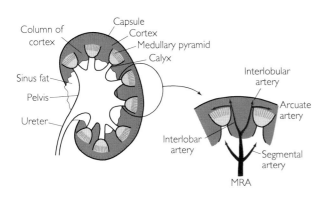

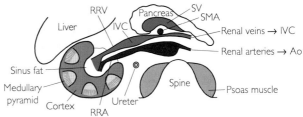

● *Key points*

1 The kidneys lie obliquely, with the left about 2 cm higher than the right.
2 The normal LS length is 9–12 cm and lengths should not differ by >2 cm in each patient.
3 The normal cortical thickness is 1.5–2.5 cm, and it thins with age.
4 The cortical echogenicity is normally slightly lower than that of the adjacent liver and spleen – mnemonic PLiSK!
5 The renal arteries arise from the aorta just inferior to the superior mesenteric artery at L2 level.

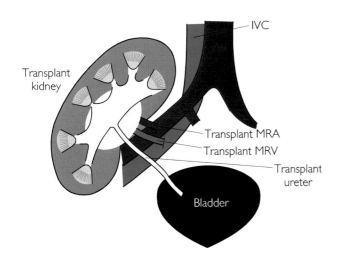

● *Key points*

1 The kidney is transplanted into either iliac fossa (more often the right).
2 There are three anastomotic sites:
   ● transplant MRA → iliac artery
   ● transplant MRV → iliac vein
   ● transplant ureter → bladder

DOI: 10.1201/9781003381655-4

PERFORMING THE SCAN

● *Step 1: Kidneys*

- **Patient position:** Supine then turn 45° to each side.
- **Preparation:** Full bladder. Empty bladder if the patient has impaired renal function.
- **Probe:** Low-frequency (3–5 MHz) curvilinear.
- **Machine:** Select renal 'preset' mode. Use two focal zones for TS imaging. Use tissue harmonics and compound imaging if the SNR is poor or with obese patients.
- **Method:** Acquire more than just representative images for each step if pathology is found.

PROBE POSITION	INSTRUCTIONS

1 LS: right kidney/liver

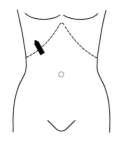

- Begin by placing the probe obliquely in the RUQ.
- Ask the patient to breathe in and hold.
- Look for the right kidney in LS and adjacent liver (if there is difficulty, try a more posterolateral approach and/or turn the patient 45° to the left).
- Compare the echogenicity of the liver parenchyma and renal cortex – the liver should be a little brighter than the kidney.
- Look for any fluid in the hepatorenal space.
- Acquire a representative image.

2 LS: right kidney

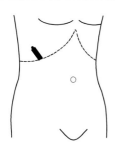

- Now turn the patient 45° onto the left side.
- Ask the patient to breathe in and hold.
- Locate the right kidney in LS again.
- Scan through the kidney in LS, observing:
  - cortical thickness and echogenicity
  - medullary pyramids
  - pelvicalyceal system
- Are there any masses, cysts, calculi or hydronephrosis?
- If rib shadows interfere, try scanning with the probe angled along a rib space.
- Measure the greatest kidney length (pole-to-pole).
- Measure any abnormalities seen.
- Acquire a representative image.

3 TS: right kidney

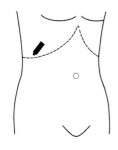

- Turn the probe 90° anticlockwise to scan in TS.
- Narrow the FOV and use two focal zones, with the second at the posterior aspect of the kidney.
- Ask the patient to breathe in and hold.
- Scan through the right kidney in TS, observing for any pathology.
- If bowel gas shadows interfere, ask the patient to push out the stomach or press over the kidney with your free hand.
- Measure any abnormalities seen.
- Acquire a representative image.

WHAT TO LOOK FOR

SCAN IMAGE

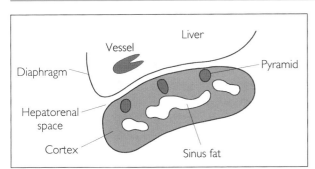

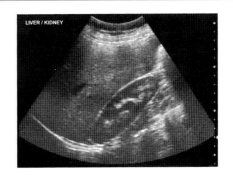

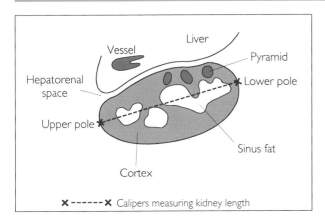

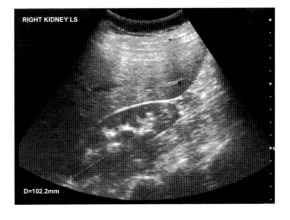

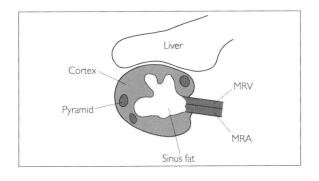

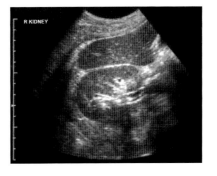

PROBE POSITION   **INSTRUCTIONS**

4 LS: left kidney/spleen

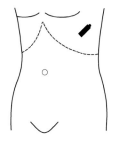

- Now turn the patient 45° onto the right side.
- Place the probe obliquely over the LUQ.
- Ask the patient to breathe in and hold.
- Look for the left kidney in LS with the spleen adjacent to it for comparison. (*Hint:* The left kidney is higher and more posterior than the right; the 11th intercostal space is a good landmark.)
- Compare the echogenicity of the spleen and the renal cortex (the spleen should be a little brighter than the kidney.
- Acquire a representative image.

5 LS: left kidney

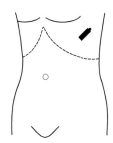

- Keep the probe in the same position.
- Scan through the left kidney in LS, observing:
  - cortical thickness and echogenicity
  - medullary pyramids
  - pelvicalyceal system
- Are there any masses, cysts, calculi or hydronephrosis?
- If rib shadows interfere, try scanning with the probe angled along a rib space.
- Measure the greatest kidney length (pole-to-pole).
- Acquire a representative image.

6 TS: left kidney

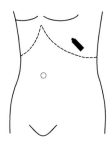

- Turn the probe 90° anticlockwise to scan in TS.
- Narrow the FOV and use two focal zones, with the second at the posterior aspect of the kidney.
- Ask the patient to breathe in and hold.
- Scan through the left kidney in TS, observing for any pathology.
- If bowel gas shadows interfere, ask the patient to push out the stomach or press over the kidney with your free hand.
- Acquire a representative image.

If a kidney cannot be found, there are three possibilities:

1 It is present but hidden – e.g. a small atrophic kidney or an abundance of bowel gas.
2 It is in an ectopic location.
3 It is absent.

Each of these should be considered in conjunction with patient history, prior investigations, etc. in order to decide.

In patients over 50 years old, it is recommended to proceed to scan the abdominal aorta and measure its calibre, looking for an aortic aneurysm (see Chapter 5).

WHAT TO LOOK FOR

SCAN IMAGE

4

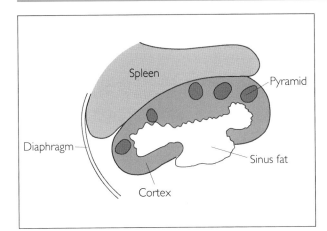

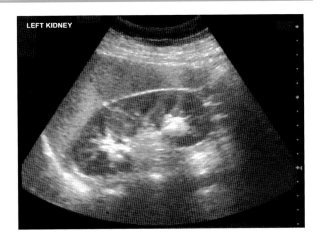

5

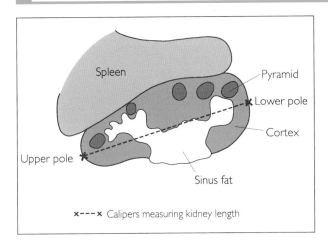

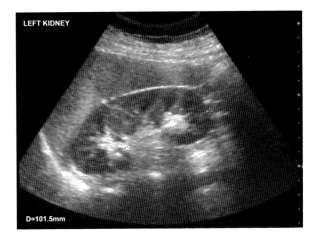

6

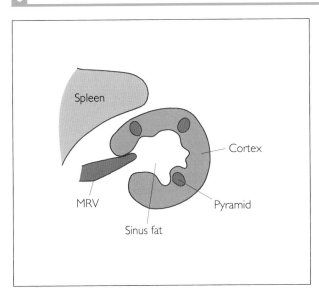

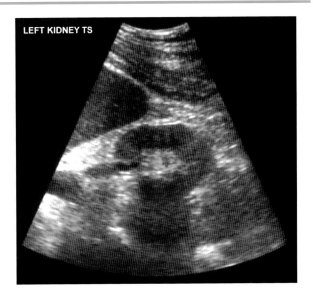

● *Step 2: Bladder*

- **Patient position:** Supine.
- **Preparation:** Full bladder. Empty bladder if the patient has impaired renal function.
- **Probe:** Low-frequency (3–5 MHz) curvilinear.
- **Machine:** It is suggested that the tissue harmonics and compound imaging be turned on. Adjust the TGC to remove reverberation artefacts from the anterior bladder wall.
- **Method:** Acquire more than just representative images for each step if pathology is found.

PROBE POSITION	INSTRUCTIONS

7 LS: bladder

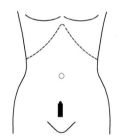

- Place the probe midline in the suprapubic area.
- Look for the bladder and adjust the depth and FOV accordingly. (*Hint:* Resting probe end on symphysis pubis often gives good views.)
- Scan across and through the bladder in LS, observing:
  - bladder wall thickness
  - bladder wall contour
  - any stones or debris?
- Acquire a representative image.
- Pitfall: Cystic pelvic masses may be mistaken for the bladder and vice versa.

8 TS: bladder

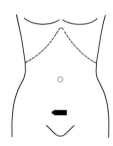

- Turn the probe 90° anticlockwise to scan in TS.
- Scan through the bladder in this plane, again looking for any pathology.
- Acquire a representative image.

9 Bladder volume

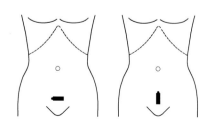

- Now calculate the bladder volume from the LS and TS images – the dual image function (split screen) is helpful for this.
- Measure the LS craniocaudal diameter.
- Measure the TS transverse and AP diameters.
- Use the measurement package to calculate the volume (on most machines): volume = A × B × C × 0.53.
- Acquire a representative image.
- Ask the patient to void, and repeat these measurement steps to calculate the postmicturition volume.

WHAT TO LOOK FOR	**SCAN IMAGE**

7

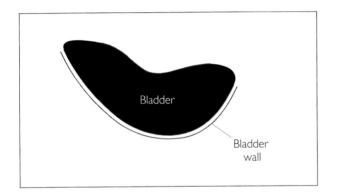

Bladder

Bladder wall

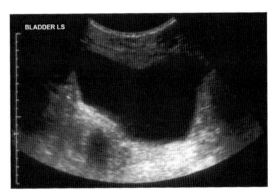

BLADDER LS

8

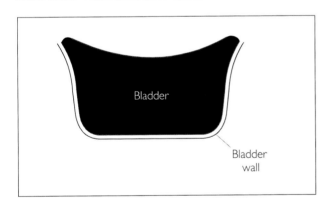

Bladder

Bladder wall

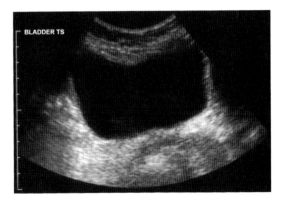

BLADDER TS

9

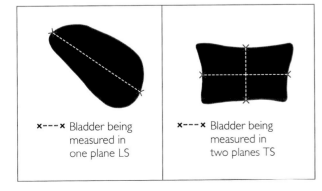

x---x Bladder being measured in one plane LS

x---x Bladder being measured in two planes TS

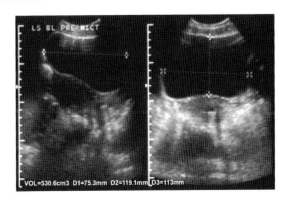

LS BL PRE MICT

VOL=530.6cm3 D1=75.3mm D2=119.1mm D3=113mm

RENAL TRANSPLANT SCAN

- **Patient position:** Supine.
- **Preparation:** Empty bladder.
- **Probe:** Low-frequency (3–5 MHz) curvilinear.
- **Machine:** Select renal preset mode. It is suggested that two focal zones are used.
- **Method:** Acquire more than just representative images for each step if pathology is found.

PROBE POSITION

INSTRUCTIONS

1 LS transplant

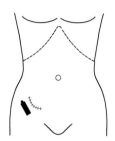

- Begin by placing the probe parallel and lateral to the iliac fossa scar (in RIF or LIF).
- Look for the transplant kidney in LS and adjust the depth and FOV accordingly.
- Scan through it in LS, then, turning the probe 90° anticlockwise, scan through it again in TS.
- Observe:
  - cortical echogenicity
  - corticomedullary differentiation
  - pelvicalyceal system dilation
  - any perirenal fluid collections?
- Acquire a representative image

Hint: If the system appears dilated check it is not due to reflux by ensuring the bladder is empty.

2 LS interlobar artery spectral Doppler

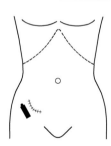

- Keep the probe in LS position.
- Turn on colour Doppler and place the colour box over the kidney.
- Optimize the colour signal: adjust the colour gain and focus position, narrow the FOV, reduce the colour box size, set the filter at low and adjust the PRF.
- Assess perfusion throughout the transplant – normally it should be to the cortical margins (power Doppler can also be used for this).
- Identify one of the interlobar arteries that run alongside the medullary pyramids.
- Turn on spectral Doppler and place the gate over this vessel, acquiring a trace. Optimize the waveform by adjusting the gate size and ensuring a beam-flow angle of 0°–60°.
- Select the calculation package (on most machines). Calculate the resistance index (RI) via the peak-systolic value S and the end-diastolic value D: $RI = (S - D)/S$.

Resistance index (RI)

1 The normal transplant has a low-resistance arterial bed with RI < 0.7
2 Higher values imply intrinsic renal disease (e.g. rejection), but cannot specify the disease type
3 It is more helpful in transplants to record serial RI values for progression over time

WHAT TO LOOK FOR

SCAN IMAGE

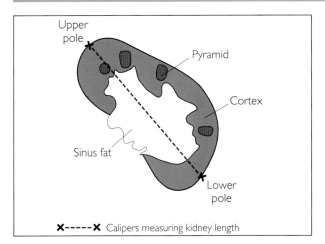

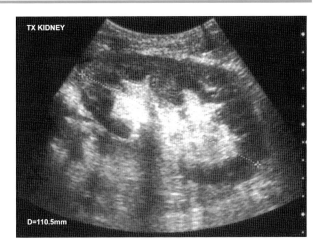

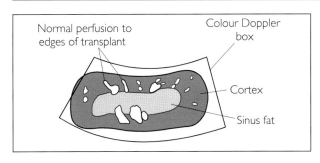

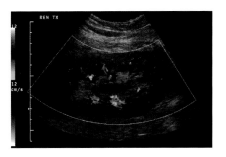

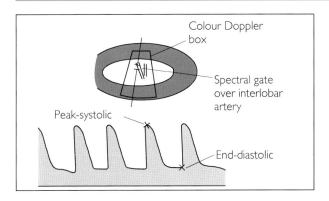

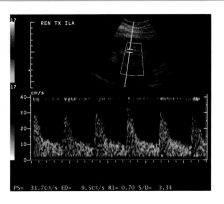

PROBE POSITION	**INSTRUCTIONS**

3 LS transplant MRA Doppler

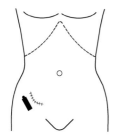

- Keep the probe in the LS position.
- Using colour Doppler, look for the MRA and MRV near the hilum, and if possible follow back to their anastomotic sites with the iliac vessels. The artery often follows a tortuous course.
- Narrow the FOV; adjust the focus and colour box size to help with this.
- Identify the MRA (flow towards probe) coming off the iliac artery. A stenosis may cause colour artefact in the adjacent soft tissues due to vibration – an ultrasound equivalent of a clinical bruit.
- Turn on spectral Doppler and place the gate over this vessel, acquiring a trace.
- Optimize the waveform by adjusting the gate size and ensuring a beam-flow angle of 0°–60°.
- Look for the normal sharp arterial systolic upstroke.
- Measure the peak-systolic flow velocity in this vessel (see below).
- Look for reverse (below baseline) end-diastolic flow on the trace – MRV thrombosis (see the pathology section for an example of this).

4 LS transplant MRV Doppler

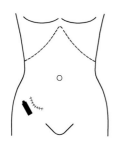

- Now identify the MRV (flow away from probe) coming off the iliac vein.
- Assess for patent flow in this vessel by acquiring a spectral Doppler trace from it.

Peak-systolic flow velocity in transplant MRA

1 Velocities > 250 cm/s are diagnostic for renal artery stenosis, which can occur at the anastomotic site
2 This is a recognized cause of graft failure and is usually treated with stenting

WHAT TO LOOK FOR

SCAN IMAGE

3a

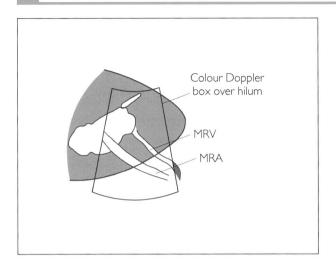

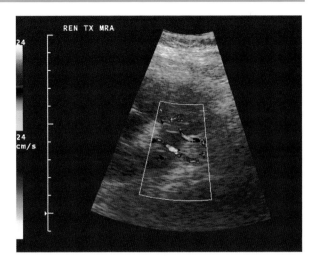

3b

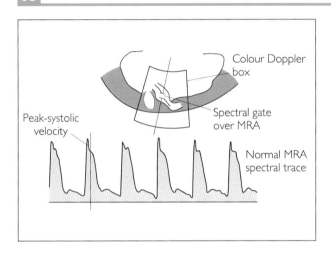

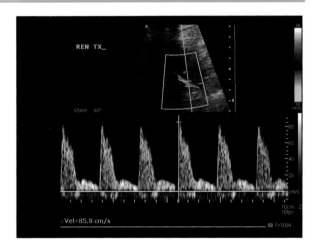

4

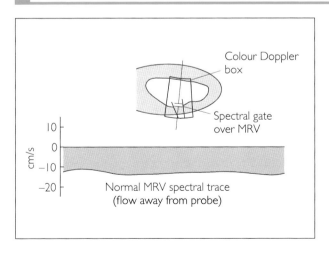

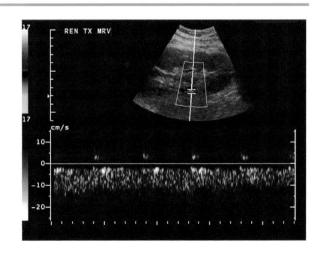

PATHOLOGY

● 1 *Congenital variants*

(a) Dromedary hump

This is a parenchymal prominence on the lateral border of the left kidney, usually just inferior to the spleen. It is important not to mistake this for a renal tumour.

(b) Column of Bertin

This is hypertrophy of a column of cortex protruding into the renal sinus fat. It is important to differentiate this from a renal tumour (continuity with the cortex the same or lower echogenicity as the cortex and normal vascularity with colour Doppler assessment).

(c) Horseshoe kidney

This is the most common renal fusion anomaly. The kidneys are connected across the midline at their lower poles by an isthmus of tissue. They are low-lying, as their normal ascent is restricted by the isthmus tethering on the inferior mesenteric artery. The lower poles are medially orientated and both renal pelvises lie anteriorly. Associated with an increased risk of stone formation, obstruction and infection, as well as certain renal tumours (e.g. Wilms' tumour).

(d) Duplex kidney

The collecting system is divided by a bridge of parenchymal tissue, with each half being drained by separate ureters. The ureter draining the upper moiety inserts into the bladder inferior and medially to the lower-moiety ureter. It is associated with a ureterocele and is prone to obstruction. The lower-moiety ureter is prone to vesico-ureteric reflux, which can lead to chronic pyelonephritis. With ultrasound, the parenchymal bridge can be difficult to see. Hydronephrosis of one moiety (usually the upper) suggests the diagnosis.

WHAT TO LOOK FOR

SCAN IMAGE

Ia Dromedary hump

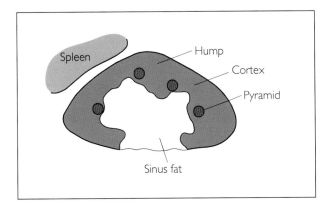

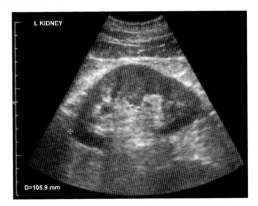

Ib Column of Bertin.

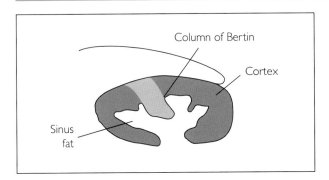

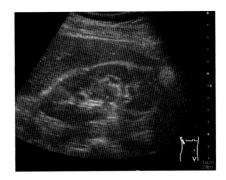

Ic Horseshoe kidney

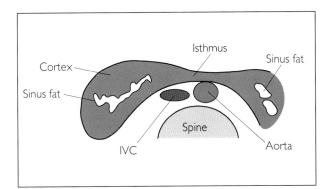

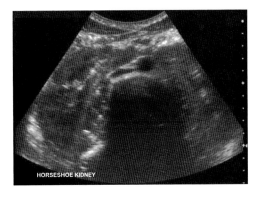

Id Duplex kidney

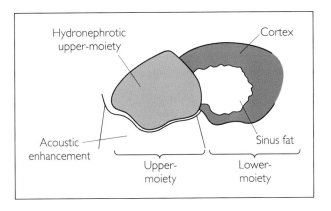

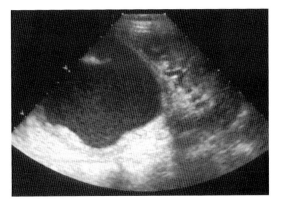

● 2 Simple renal cysts

These are a very common finding, increasing in frequency with age. They are most commonly located in the cortex.

Ultrasound features
- Smooth edge
- Thin wall
- Echo-free contents (may contain a few fine septations)
- Post-acoustic enhancement

Hint: Any cyst with atypical features (thick or multiple septations, solid components, wall nodularity) requires CT or MRI assessment and consideration of surgical excision.

● 3 Adult polycystic kidney disease (PCKD)

In this autosomal dominant condition, the kidneys contain multiple numbers of cysts, which slowly enlarge, causing cortical thinning and progressive renal failure. The cysts may be visible on ultrasound by the second decade but usually remain asymptomatic until mid-40s.

Ultrasound features
- The kidneys are enlarged, with an undulating surface
- They contain multiple cysts of varying sizes
- The cysts are typically simple but some may have a more complex appearance due to internal haemorrhage

Look for associated cysts in the liver (50%), pancreas (10%) and spleen (rare).

Age-related diagnostic criteria for adult PCKD (in someone with a family history of PCKD)
1. Age 15–30: at least two unilateral or bilateral renal cysts
2. Age 31–59: at least two cysts in each kidney
3. Age >60: at least four cysts in each kidney

● 4 Renal stones (nephrolithiasis)

Calcium containing stones are the most common type. Patients are often asymptomatic, but may suffer recurrent urinary tract infections or bouts of renal colic.

Ultrasound features
- Echo-bright focus that casts a distal acoustic shadow
- May be difficult to detect if obscured by renal sinus echoes
- If a stone has caused ureteric obstruction, then hydronephrosis may be seen

Hint: Always measure the size of any stones and note their location.

Hint: Increasing the frequency and reducing the overall gain makes stone detection easier.

WHAT TO LOOK FOR   **SCAN IMAGE**

2 Simple renal cyst

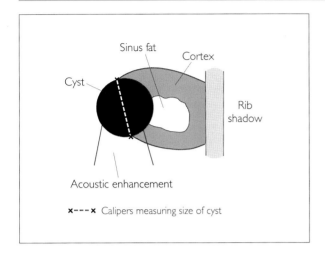

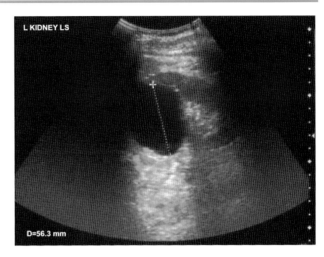

3 Adult PCKD

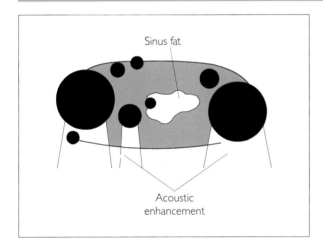

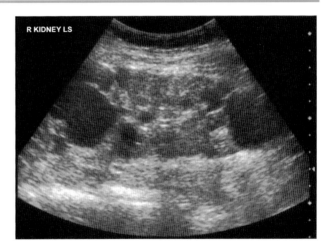

4 Renal stones

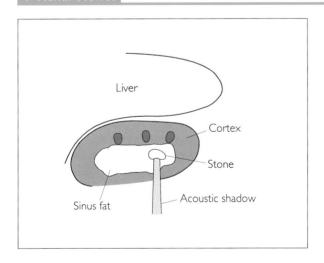

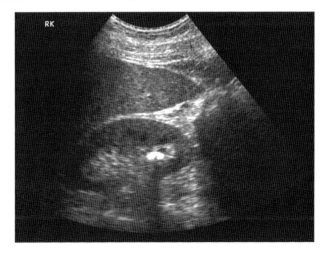

● 5 Hydronephrosis

This is obstructive dilation of the collecting system; most commonly caused by a stone, tumour or blood clot. It can be graded as follows:

(a) Mild

There is separation of renal sinus echoes – the 'split sinus' sign. This should be differentiated from back-pressure effects of a full bladder by rescanning the patient after they have voided; the system should decompress within a few minutes. It should also be differentiated from prominent renal vessels by using colour Doppler.

(b) Moderate

The pelvis and calyces are swollen, but there is no loss of cortical thickness.

(c) Severe

The system is grossly swollen, with loss of sinus fat echoes and cortical thinning.

WHAT TO LOOK FOR

SCAN IMAGE

5a Mild hydronephrosis

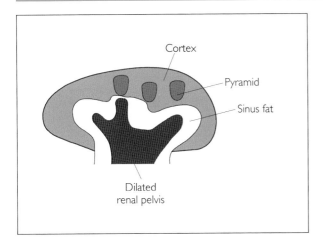

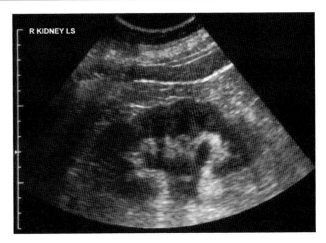

5b Moderate hydronephrosis

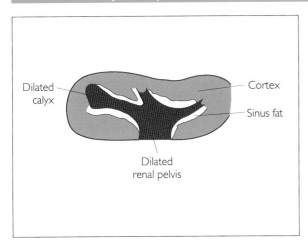

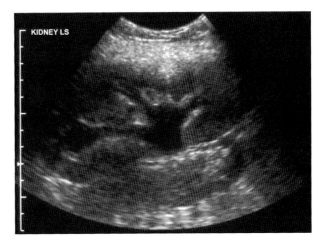

5c Severe hydronephrosis

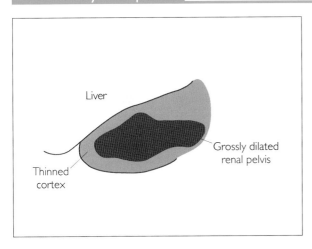

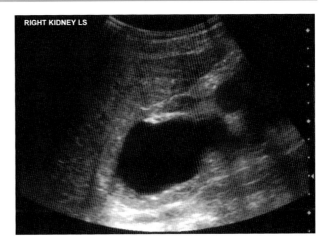

● 6 *Angiomyolipoma*

This is a benign mixed tumour of blood vessels, muscle and fat. It tends to enlarge with age and is more common in females.

Ultrasound features

- Cortical-based lesion
- Usually a small (<2 cm) sharply defined echo-bright mass
- One-third will cast a post-acoustic shadow
- Multiple bilateral lesions may be seen in tuberous sclerosis patients

Hint: The main differential diagnosis for angiomyolipoma is a milk of calcium cyst and small parenchymal stone. Larger angiomyolipomas (>3 cm) can mimic the appearance of a small renal cell carcinoma CT characterization is recommended for lesions >1.5 cm to ensure they contain fat. Serial ultrasound follow-up is recommended for lesions <1.5 cm to ensure stability. Large AMLs have a recognized risk of spontaneous haemorrhage.

● 7 *Renal cell carcinoma (RCC)*

This is the most common renal malignancy in adults.

Ultrasound features

- Mass, usually of mixed echogenicity, often causing bulging of the renal contour
- Small tumours can be echo-bright and look similar to angiomyolipomas

It is important to assess the renal vein and inferior vena cava for tumour thrombus. The other kidney should also be inspected carefully, as 5% are bilateral.

WHAT TO LOOK FOR   **SCAN IMAGE**

6 Small angiomyolipoma

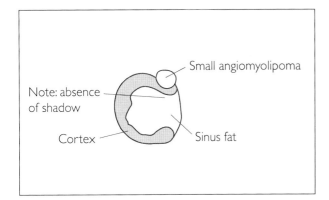

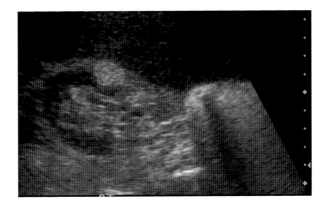

7 RCC

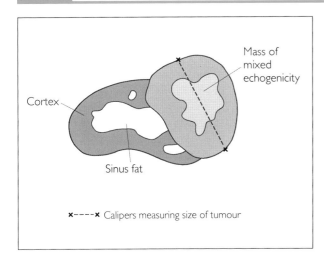

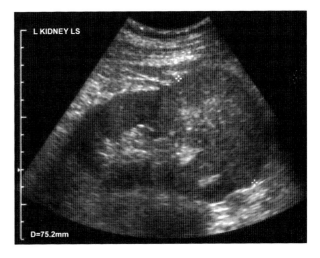

● 8 Renal artery stenosis (RAS)

This presents clinically as resistant hypertension. The majority of cases are caused by atherosclerosis, which tends to involve the proximal portion of the MRA. Rarely, it is due to fibromuscular dysplasia, which affects the MRA more distally. RAS is thought to be clinically significant only if the stenosis is >70%.

Ultrasound features
- Unilateral small kidney (>2 cm size difference)
- Interlobar artery spectral Doppler shows loss of the normal sharp systolic upstroke. It has a dampened, rounded 'parvus tardus' waveform with acceleration time (AT) >0.07 s and more specifically >0.12 s.
- The MRA has a peak-systolic velocity over 180 cm/s.

Hint: Doppler ultrasound has a low sensitivity for RAS, i.e., it cannot reliably exclude the diagnosis, and further imaging with CT/MRI or catheter angiography is required.

● 9 Renal failure

(a) Acute renal failure

There is significant deterioration of renal function over hours–days.

- **Prerenal:** caused by hypoperfusion.
- **Renal:** causes include acute glomerulonephritis and acute tubular necrosis (e.g. contrast reaction).
- **Postrenal:** due to outflow obstruction (e.g. ovarian malignancy, ureteric stone).

Ultrasound features
Prerenal/renal
- Kidneys are usually of normal size
- Renal cortex may be echo-bright and/or swollen
- Pyramids can appear prominent: 'punched-out pyramids' sign
- Interlobar artery RI is usually raised

Postrenal
- Look for hydronephrosis (see earlier)

(b) Chronic renal failure

There is long-standing loss of renal function over months–years. Causes include chronic glomerulonephritis and diabetic/hypertensive nephropathy.

Ultrasound features
- Kidneys are small (it may be impossible to find them)
- Renal cortex is thinned and echo-bright

WHAT TO LOOK FOR **SCAN IMAGE**

8 RAS

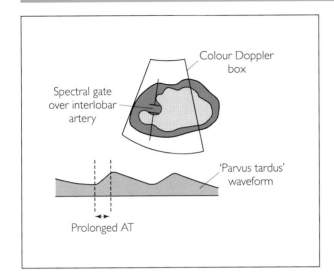

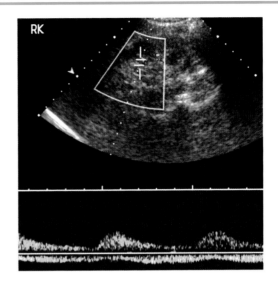

9a Acute renal failure

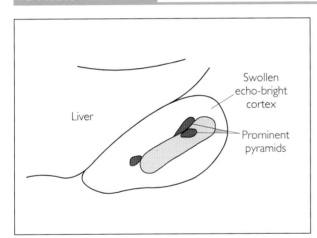

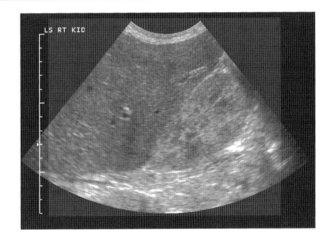

9b Chronic renal failure

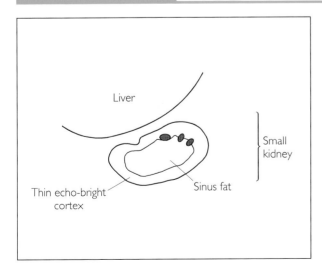

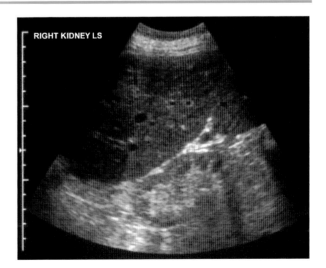

● 10 Pyelonephritis

This is a urinary tract infection involving the kidney, either by migration up the ureter or via hematogenous seeding. The renal pelvis and parenchyma become inflamed. Ultrasound is mainly used to assess for predisposing factors to infection, e.g. congenital anomalies, calculi, as well as complications such as abscess formation and hydronephrosis.

Ultrasound features
- Commonly normal with no visible abnormality (up to 75% of cases)

Positive findings include:

- Echo-poor areas (oedema)
- Echo-bright areas (haemorrhage)
- Mixed echogenicity areas (oedema and haemorrhage)
- Loss of corticomedullary differentiation
- Multiple small echo-free foci suggest micro-abscesses
- Focal pyelonephritis typically appears as a wedge-shaped focus of mixed echogenicity with diminished blood flow on colour Doppler assessment

● 11 Renal infarct

This is a severe ischaemic event causing the death of a segment of renal parenchyma. Causes include:

- embolism: infective endocarditis, post-myocardial infarction mural thrombus
- thrombosis: vasculitis, sickle cell disease crisis
- trauma: causing injury to the main renal artery

Ultrasound features
- Echo-bright wedge-shaped cortical defect over the site of a renal pyramid. Similar apparent defects lying between pyramids are usually due to congenital foetal lobulation.

WHAT TO LOOK FOR   **SCAN IMAGE**

10 Pyelonephritis

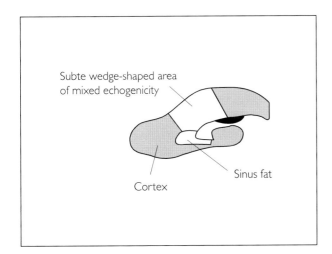

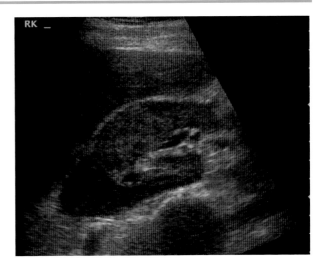

11 Renal infarct

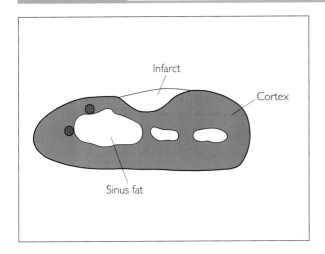

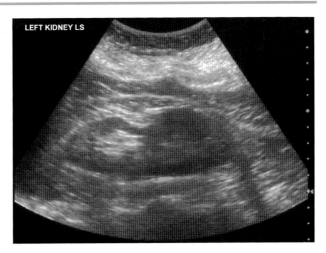

● 12 Bladder wall thickening

The bladder needs to be well-distended for accurate assessment. Wall thickness >5 mm is abnormal. Chronic bacterial cystitis and ketamine abuse are well-recognized causes of generalized thickening.

A focal thickening may be due to a bladder cancer (e.g. TCC) and must be distinguished from a hematoma – cancers will not move on patient re-positioning and may display internal blood flow with colour Doppler.

● 13 Ureterocele

This is a cystic dilation of the distal ureter at its bladder insertion. There is a strong association with duplex kidneys, where the ureter draining the upper moiety tends to be the one involved. Ureteroceles can cause ureteric obstruction, and stones may form within them.

Ultrasound features
- Thin-walled cystic projection at the site of ureteric insertion
- Always look for any associated obstruction (hydroureter or hydronephrosis)

WHAT TO LOOK FOR **SCAN IMAGE**

12a Bladder wall thickening

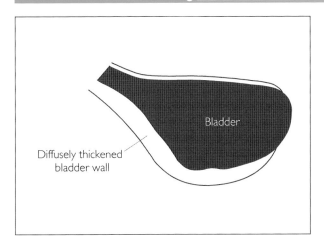

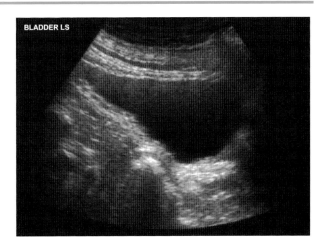

12b Bladder carcinoma

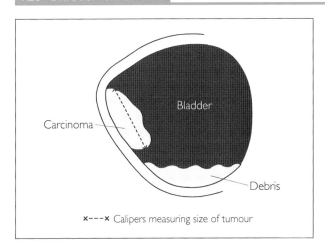

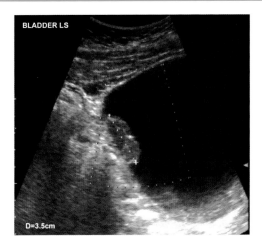

13 Ureterocele

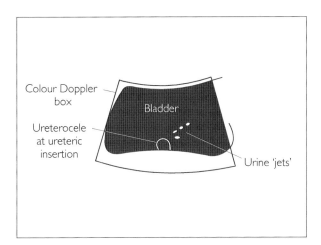

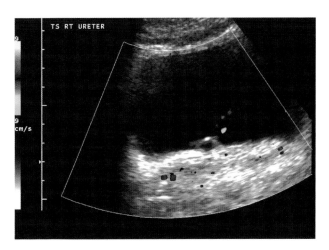

● 14 Transplant kidney fluid collections

Collections of blood, lymph and urine around the transplant are very common in the postoperative period. Most are incidental findings and resolve spontaneously. However, occasionally they can be large and compress the graft, impairing its function. These may then need drainage.

Ultrasound features
Lymphocele
- Commonest collection
- Occurs weeks to months post operation
- Seen as an echo-free area that classically has internal septations

Hematoma
- Occurs immediately post operation
- In early stages, seen as an echo-free area
- May later contain echo-bright fibrin strands

Urinoma
- Uncommon collection
- Occurs early post operation
- Seen as an echo-free area

Ultrasound cannot usually distinguish between these different collections; however, it has a role to play in monitoring their regression. Rarely, a collection may become infected, leading to abscess formation.

● 15 Transplant rejection (acute)

This is mediated via cellular immunity. It occurs most commonly during the first month post operation. The patient is systemically unwell, with a tender swollen graft.

Ultrasound features
- Swollen kidney
- Echo-bright renal cortex
- Reduced brightness of renal sinus fat
- Interlobar artery spectral Doppler RI > 0.7

These features are also seen in acute tubular necrosis and cyclosporine toxicity, and they should be considered in conjunction with the patient history. Serial RI values may help but often a biopsy is needed to establish the diagnosis.

WHAT TO LOOK FOR   **SCAN IMAGE**

14a Post-transplant lymphocele

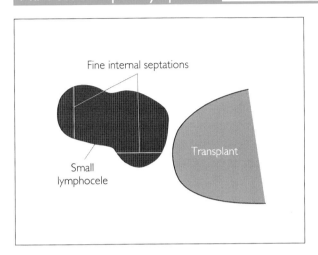

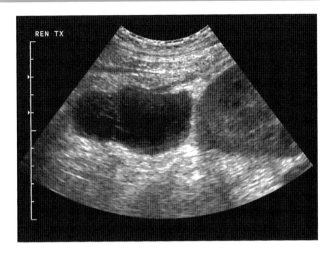

14b Post-transplant urinoma

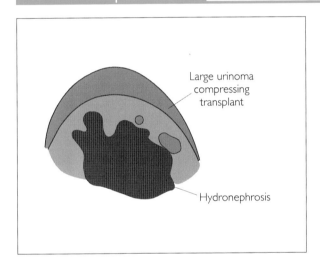

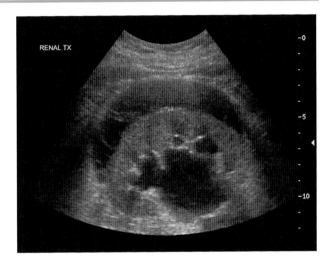

15 Transplant rejection (acute)

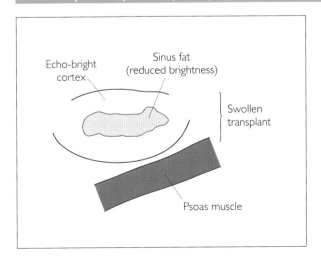

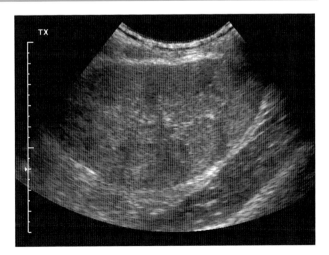

● *16 Transplant kidney main renal vein (MRV) thrombosis*

This is a rare, but serious, early complication. The patient will be oliguric, with a tender, swollen graft.

Ultrasound features
- Swollen kidney with subcapsular fluid collections
- Reduced cortical perfusion
- Note the absence of flow in the MRV
- Look for the characteristic MRA waveform, which shows reverse end-diastolic flow

The transplant is non-viable and must be removed.

WHAT TO LOOK FOR

SCAN IMAGE

16 Transplant kidney MRV thrombosis

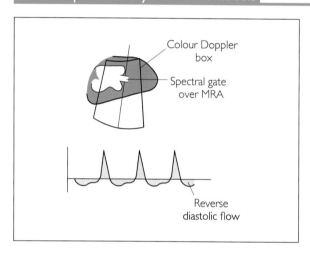

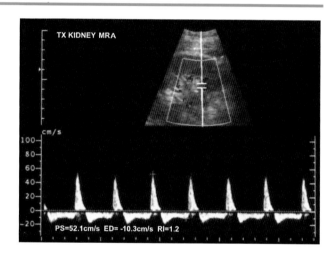

PS=52.1cm/s ED= -10.3cm/s RI=1.2

Abdominal aorta

ANATOMY

Anterior view of abdominal aorta

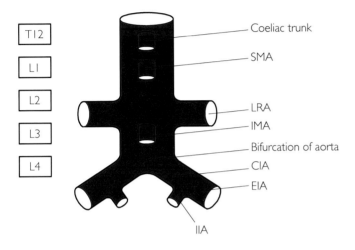

T12
L1
L2
L3
L4

Coeliac trunk
SMA
LRA
IMA
Bifurcation of aorta
CIA
EIA
IIA

Transverse section of renal arteries and aorta

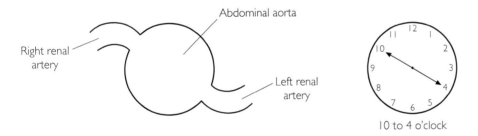

Abdominal aorta
Right renal artery
Left renal artery

10 to 4 o'clock

In the TS section, the renal arteries are seen to branch off the aorta at the 10 to 4 o'clock positions.

● Key points

1 The main branches of the aorta exit at the following vertebral levels:

	Approximate vertebral level
Coeliac trunk	T12
SMA	L1
Renal arteries	L2/3
IMA	L3
Bifurcation of aorta	L4

2 Normal diameter of abdominal aorta <2 cm.
3 Normal diameter of common iliac arteries <1 cm.

DOI: 10.1201/9781003381655-5

PERFORMING THE SCAN

- **Patient position:** Supine.
- **Preparation:** Nil by mouth for 8 hours.
- **Probe:** Low-frequency (3–5 MHz) curvilinear.
- **Machine:** Select the abdomen preset mode. Set the focus on the posterior wall of the aorta. Use tissue harmonics and compound imaging if the SNR is poor or with obese patients.
- **Method:** Start at the upper abdomen and scan caudally in at least two planes. Acquire more than one representative image for each step if pathology is found.

PROBE POSITION

INSTRUCTIONS

1 TS: upper abdominal aorta

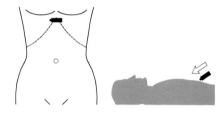

- Place the probe just inferior to the xiphisternum and angle it cranially. Look for the 'seagull sign' of the coeliac trunk at T12 level. The body of the 'seagull' is the coeliac trunk and the wings are the hepatic and splenic arteries branching off.
- Acquire representative image(s).

2 TS: aorta

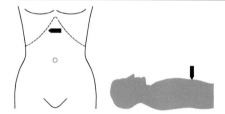

- Now angle the probe so that it is perpendicular to the abdomen and scan caudally, following the course of the aorta until it bifurcates. Look for any irregularities in the vessel wall.
- Measure the maximum inner to inner AP diameter in TS of the suprarenal aorta and infrarenal aorta at its widest point.
- The renal arteries are difficult to visualize directly. To locate the region of the renal arteries, first look for the 'tadpole sign' of the portal confluence/splenic vein, then look posterior to this to find the SMA. The renal arteries arise 1 cm caudal to the SMA origin.
- Acquire representative image(s).

3 Colour Doppler TS: aorta

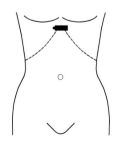

- Place the probe just inferior to the xiphisternum again. Turn on colour Doppler and place the colour box over the aorta.
- Optimize the colour signal: adjust the colour gain and focus position, narrow the sector width, reduce the colour box size, and set the PRF at high and the filter at medium.
- Scan caudally, following the course of the aorta until it bifurcates. Look for any filling defects.
- Acquire representative image(s).

WHAT TO LOOK FOR

SCAN IMAGE

1

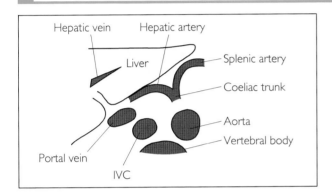

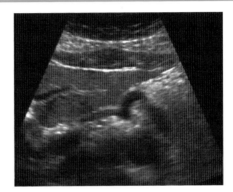

2

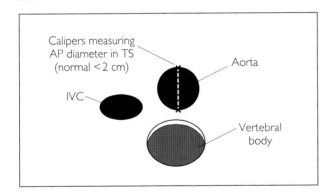

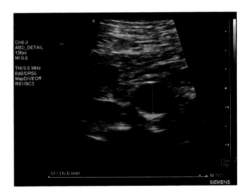

3

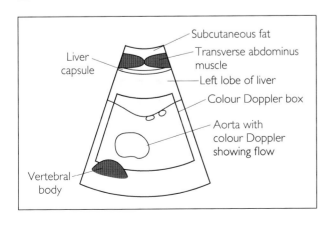

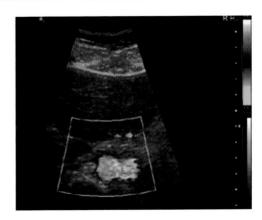

PROBE POSITION	**INSTRUCTIONS**

4 LS: aorta

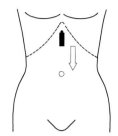

- Return to the xiphisternum and locate the upper abdominal aorta in TS as in Step 1.
- Rotate the probe through 90° clockwise so that the aorta is now imaged in LS.
- Follow the course of the aorta caudally in LS until it bifurcates. Look for any vessel wall irregularities.
- Look specifically for the origin of the SMA: just posterior to this the LRV should be visible, and it should be possible to describe any anomalies in relation to the renal vessels. The distance from the SMA to any aneurysm should be measured and documented.
- If there is difficulty in following the aorta in LS, try a coronal view instead – i.e. place the probe in the left flank and angle it towards the vertebral column.
- Measure the maximum inner to inner AP diameter in LS of the suprarenal or infrarenal aorta at its widest point.
- Acquire representative image(s).

5 Colour Doppler LS: aorta

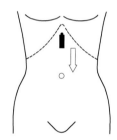

- Now turn on colour Doppler and place the colour box over the aorta.
- Optimize the colour signal: adjust the gain and focus position, narrow the FOV, reduce the colour box size, and set the PRF at high and the filter at medium. Doppler angle should be 0°–60° to demonstrate flow. Heel-toe the probe to facilitate obtaining a good Doppler angle with the aorta.
- Repeat Step 4, looking for any filling defects.
- Acquire representative image(s).

6 Common iliac arteries

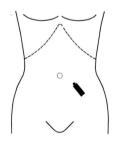

- Turn off colour Doppler. Place the probe over the bifurcation of the aorta in TS, then follow each CIA caudally as far as possible, looking for any vessel wall irregularities.
- Measure the maximum AP diameter of each CIA in TS but if this proves too difficult measure approximately in LS.
- Turn on colour Doppler and repeat this step, looking for any filling defects.
- Return the probe to the bifurcation of the aorta in TS. Rotate the probe through 90° clockwise and now scan each CIA in LS with and without colour Doppler.
- Acquire representative image(s).

WHAT TO LOOK FOR

SCAN IMAGE

4

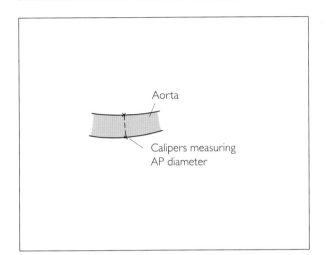

Aorta

Calipers measuring
AP diameter

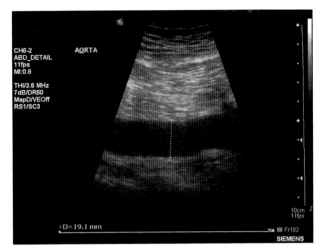

5

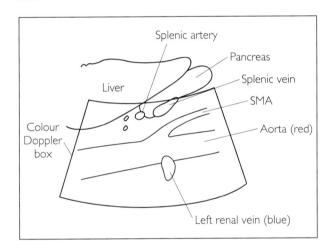

Splenic artery

Pancreas

Splenic vein

Liver

SMA

Colour
Doppler
box

Aorta (red)

Left renal vein (blue)

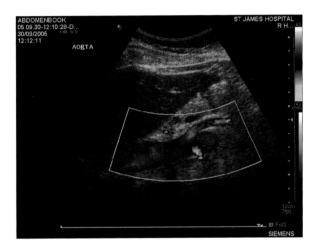

6

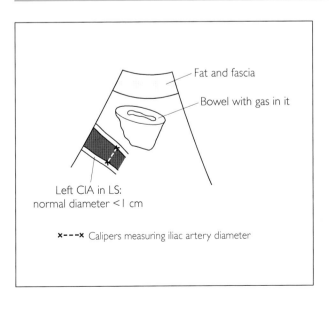

Fat and fascia

Bowel with gas in it

Left CIA in LS:
normal diameter <1 cm

x---x Calipers measuring iliac artery diameter

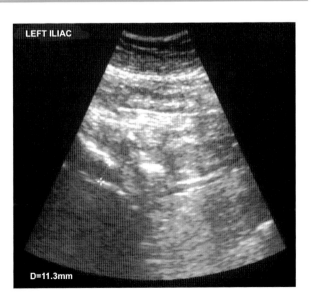

ABDOMINAL AORTA: COMMON PATHOLOGY

● *1 Aneurysm*

An aneurysm is a localized dilation of an artery by at least 50% (<50% = ectasia) compared with the normal diameter of the vessel. Aneurysms occur in 5% of patients >65 years old. Major risk factors are atherosclerosis, age and inflammation (e.g. malignancy, syphilis).

Ultrasound features

Localized dilatation of artery: measure AP diameter in TS and LS inner wall to the inner wall.

Diameter (cm)	Description	Risk of rupture per year	Action
<2	Normal		Nil
2.5–2.9	Ectatic		Nil
3.0–4.4	Low-risk aneurysm	1% per year	Monitor 12 monthly
4.5–5.4	Low-risk aneurysm	1% per year	Monitor 3 monthly
>5.5	High-risk aneurysm	5% per year	Refer to vascular team
>7	High-risk aneurysm	>25% per year	Refer urgently to the vascular team.

Note: If the patient has any symptoms related to the aneurysm – e.g. abdominal/back pain, collapse, etc. (regardless of the size of the aneurysm) – discuss with the vascular team on the same day.

● *2 Atheromatous plaques*

Atherosclerosis is a disease of large- and medium-sized muscular arteries. It is characterized by the accumulation of lipids, calcium and cellular debris within the intima of the vessel wall, forming atheromatous plaques. These plaques result in luminal obstruction, abnormalities of blood flow and diminished oxygen supply to target organs. The major risk factors are smoking, hypercholesterolaemia, diabetes and hypertension.

Ultrasound features

- Localized irregular thickening of the vessel wall (measured in TS and LS)
- The echogenicity of the plaque depends on its contents:
  - echo-poor: blood- or lipid-filled = increased risk of rupture
  - echo-bright: calcified = more benign
- Filling defects with colour Doppler
- Classify using a modified Gray–Weale classification; see page 142. [AC Grey Weale et al. *J Cardiovasc Surg* 1988; 29: 676–81]

WHAT TO LOOK FOR

SCAN IMAGE

1a Aneurysmal aorta

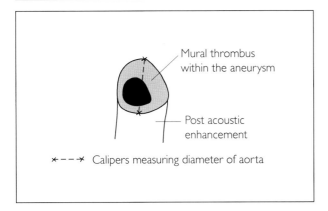

Mural thrombus within the aneurysm

Post acoustic enhancement

✶– – –✶ Calipers measuring diameter of aorta

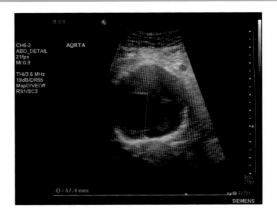

1b Ectatic aorta

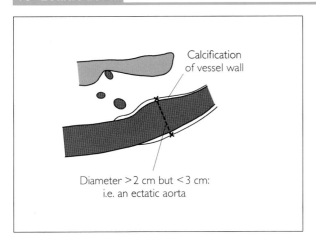

Calcification of vessel wall

Diameter >2 cm but <3 cm: i.e. an ectatic aorta

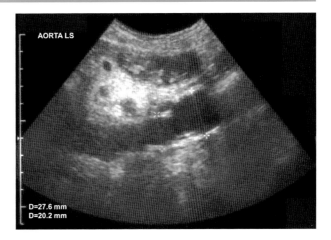

2 Atheromatous plaques

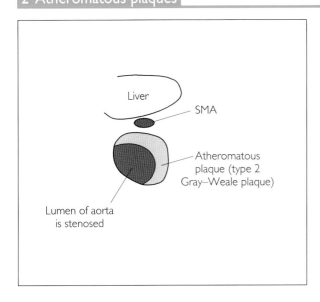

Liver

SMA

Atheromatous plaque (type 2 Gray–Weale plaque)

Lumen of aorta is stenosed

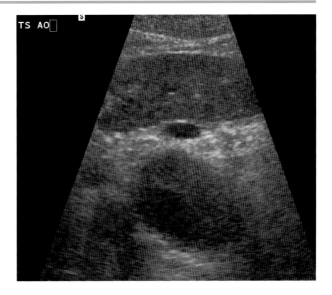

6 Liver transplant

PRE-TRANSPLANT: INDICATIONS FOR SCAN

There are two groups of patients for whom the preoperative liver transplant protocol should be performed: those who are known to have chronic liver disease and are being considered for the transplant waiting list and those who have evidence of chronic liver disease on ultrasound and may potentially require a transplant in the future.

The indications for liver transplantation are as follows:

1 Cirrhosis from chronic liver disease:
   - hepatitis
   - alcoholic liver disease
   - primary biliary cirrhosis
   - primary sclerosing cholangitis
   - Wilson's disease
   - hemochromatosis
   - Budd–Chiari syndrome
2 Fulminant hepatic failure – e.g. paracetamol overdose or acute hepatitis.
3 Congenital liver failure:
   - polycystic disease
   - Caroli's disease
4 Hepatocellular carcinoma (HCC).

PRE-TRANSPLANT: MAIN AIMS OF SCAN

1 Confirm the initial diagnosis (if there is one).
2 Assess vessel patency and any associated complications.
3 Assess any contraindications to transplant:
   - extrahepatic malignancy
   - systemic sepsis
   - cholangiocarcinoma
   - porto–superior mesenteric vein thrombosis
   - HCC >5 cm or >3 HCC tumours

DOI: 10.1201/9781003381655-6

PRE-TRANSPLANT: PERFORMING THE SCAN

- **Patient position:** Supine.
- **Preparation:** Clear fluid only for 8 hours.
- **Probe:** Low-frequency (3–5 MHz) curvilinear.
- **Machine:** Select abdomen preset mode.
- **Method:**
  (a) Full abdomen protocol, looking specifically for cirrhosis, ascites, splenomegaly and varices.
  (b) Perform Doppler examination of hepatic artery, hepatic veins, portal vein, splenic vein and inferior vena cava.

PROBE POSITION

INSTRUCTIONS

1 Liver

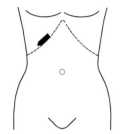

- Place the probe in the RUQ and scan through the liver in at least two planes.
- It is often difficult to clearly image a shrunken cirrhotic liver. Therefore ask the patient to take deep breaths in as the probe is angled caudally under the subcostal margin Or try an intercostal approach. Turning the patient on their side may help.
- Examine the liver, taking note of:
  – any focal lesions, metastases, HCC?
  – echogenicity: diffuse and focal
  – echotexture: coarse?
  – size: is it shrunken and cirrhotic?
  – surface: is it nodular or smooth?
  – ducts: are they dilated?
- Examine the subphrenic and subhepatic spaces. Look specifically for ascites.
- Acquire representative images.

2 Complete abdomen protocol scan

- See Chapter 3 for details.
- Pay particular attention to the following:
  – CBD: measure diameter
  – spleen: is there splenomegaly?
  – any contraindications to transplant?
- Acquire representative images.

WHAT TO LOOK FOR

SCAN IMAGE

1

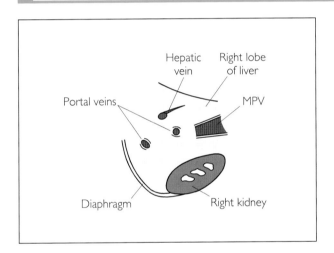

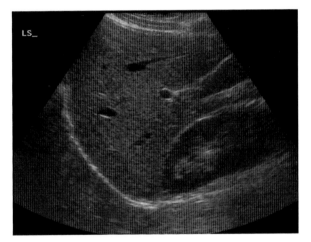

2

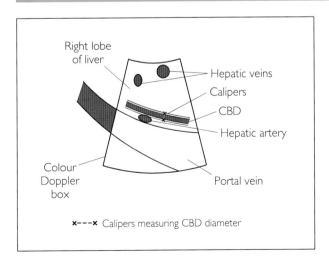

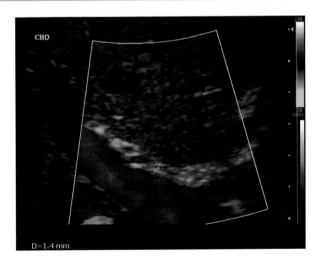

PROBE POSITION

INSTRUCTIONS

3 Main hepatic artery spectral Doppler

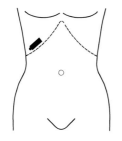

- Place the probe in the RUQ intercostally. The position varies between patients, but try the 11th ICS AAL or MCL. Find the portal vein and then look anterior to it to visualize the MHA.
- Turn on colour Doppler. Optimize the colour signal: adjust the colour gain and focus position, narrow the FOV, reduce the colour box size, and set the PRF at medium and the filter at medium.
- Take note of flow in the hepatic artery. If no flow is detected, turn up the colour gain and reduce the PRF scale. Change the Doppler frequency to its lowest setting or change to a lower frequency probe. If still no flow is detected, the hepatic artery may be occluded. Consider if contrast medium enhancement is appropriate.
- If flow is detected, turn on spectral Doppler and place the gate over the hepatic artery, acquiring a trace. Optimize the waveform by adjusting the gate size and ensuring a beam-flow angle of 0°–60°.
- *Hint:* Ask the patient to breathe gently or hold their breath to aid measurement.
- Select the calculation package. Calculate the acceleration time (AT) via the interval from end-diastole to the first peak of the systolic upstroke. Calculate the resistance index (RI) via the peak-systolic value S and the trough diastolic value D: $RI = (S - D)/S$.
- Normal values are RI >0.5 and AT <0.08 s.
- Acquire representative image(s).

4 Main portal vein spectral Doppler

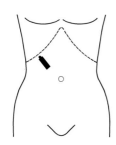

- Find the portal vein by placing the probe perpendicular to the right costal margin MCL.
- Turn on colour Doppler and assess patency.
- Turn on spectral Doppler and place the gate over the portal vein, acquiring a trace. Optimize the waveform by adjusting the gate size and ensuring a beam-flow angle of 60° or less. Measure the peak velocity and record the direction and character of flow.
- Normal peak velocity = 16–40 cm/s.
- Normal direction: hepatopetal.
- Normal character: alters with respiration; may have transmitted pulsation from IVC in a slim patient.
- Acquire representative image(s).

WHAT TO LOOK FOR

SCAN IMAGE

3

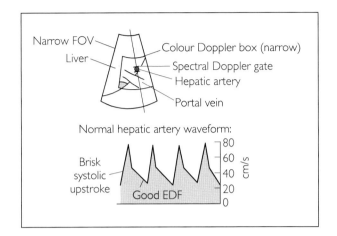

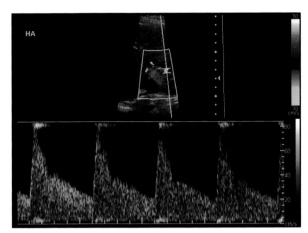

4

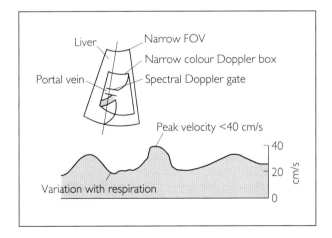

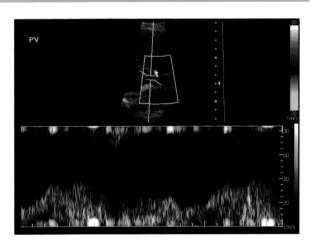

PROBE POSITION	INSTRUCTIONS

5 Hepatic veins spectral Doppler

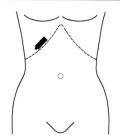

- To examine the hepatic veins, place the probe parallel to the right costal margin and angle it caudally under the costal margin as the patient inspires. If there is difficulty finding the hepatic veins, try an intercostal approach.
- Turn on colour Doppler and optimize the colour signal as described in Step 1.
- Assess the patency of all three hepatic veins.
- Turn on spectral Doppler and place the gate over a hepatic vein, acquiring a trace. Optimize the waveform by adjusting the gate size.
- The normal waveform is a classical triphasic pattern and varies with respiration.
- Acquire representative image(s).

6 IVC spectral Doppler

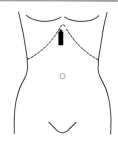

- To image the IVC, place the probe LS inferior to the xiphisternum and just right of the midline.
- Alternatively, place the probe in the right MCL and angle it towards the left flank.
- Turn on colour Doppler to assess patency.
- Turn on spectral Doppler and place the gate over the IVC, acquiring a trace. Optimize the waveform by adjusting the gate size.
- Normal flow is pulsatile with reverse flow during right atrial systole; it varies with respiration.
- Acquire representative image(s).

7 Splenic vein spectral Doppler

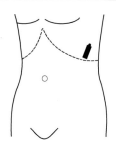

- Ask the patient to turn 45° onto the right side.
- Place the probe in the left 11th ICS AAL to image the spleen. Measure the spleen length.
- Turn on colour Doppler and locate the splenic vein. Is it patent? Are there any varices? Follow the course of the splenic vein posterior to the pancreas.
- Turn on spectral Doppler and place the gate over the splenic vein, acquiring a trace. Optimize the waveform by adjusting the gate size and ensuring a beam-flow angle of 0°–60°.
- Normal flow is hepatopetal/away from the probe and varies with respiration.
- Acquire representative image(s).

WHAT TO LOOK FOR

SCAN IMAGE

5

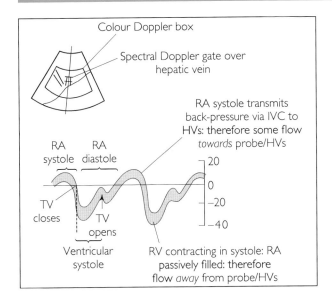

Colour Doppler box

Spectral Doppler gate over hepatic vein

RA systole | RA diastole

TV closes | TV opens

Ventricular systole

RA systole transmits back-pressure via IVC to HVs: therefore some flow *towards* probe/HVs

RV contracting in systole: RA passively filled: therefore flow *away* from probe/HVs

20
0
−20
−40

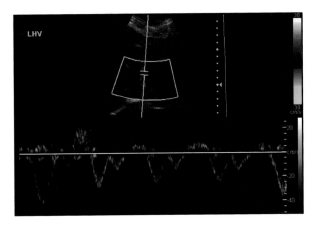

6

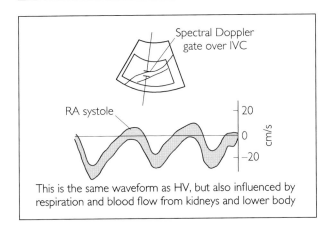

Spectral Doppler gate over IVC

RA systole

20
0
−20

cm/s

This is the same waveform as HV, but also influenced by respiration and blood flow from kidneys and lower body

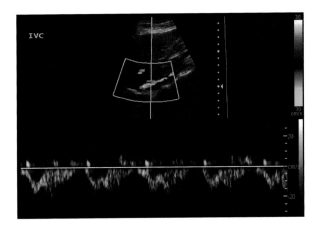

7

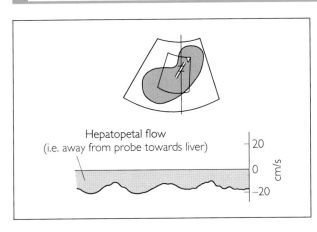

Hepatopetal flow
(i.e. away from probe towards liver)

20
0
−20

cm/s

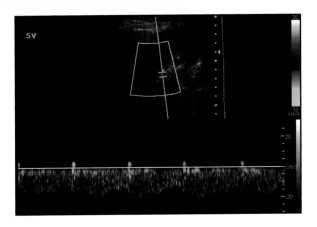

PRE-TRANSPLANT: PATHOLOGY

Refer also to the hepatobiliary pathology section in Chapter 3.

● 1 Portal hypertension

Increased pressure in the portal venous system results in blood from the gut bypassing the liver via collateral veins. These veins then dilate and form varices. The most common causes are cirrhosis, alcoholic hepatitis and portal vein thrombosis.

Ultrasound features

● Portal vein flow varies with the severity of hypertension:

Degree of portal hypertension	Spectral Doppler waveform
Very mild	Loss of variation with respiration
Mild	Slowed peak velocity, i.e. <10 cm/s
Moderate	Balanced, i.e. forward and reverse flow together
Severe	Reversed flow
Complete occlusion	No flow

● Hepatic artery may show increased flow (compensating for reduced flow into the liver from the portal vein)
● Associated features:
 − ascites
 − varices
 − splenomegaly
 − recanalized umbilical vein

● 2 Portal vein thrombosis

Thrombosis may cause complete or partial occlusion of the vein. The most common causes are cirrhosis, pancreatitis and gastrointestinal malignancy. HCC may result in tumour thrombus in the portal vein, and arterial flow may be seen within the portal vein due to neo-angiogenesis (with colour Doppler).

Two to three weeks after a portal vein is thrombosed, a mass of tortuous vessels may form at the porta hepatis. This is called cavernous transformation and may be mistaken for biliary dilation unless colour and spectral Doppler are used to identify flow in the vessels.

Ultrasound features
● Fresh thrombus: echo-free
● 4-hour-old thrombus: low-level echoes
● Cavernous transformation (see above)
● Colour Doppler: a filling defect if thrombosis causes stenosis
● Colour Doppler: no flow if the thrombosis causes occlusion
● Spectral Doppler: increased velocity at stenosis site

WHAT TO LOOK FOR   **SCAN IMAGE**

1a Portal hypertension (mild/moderate)

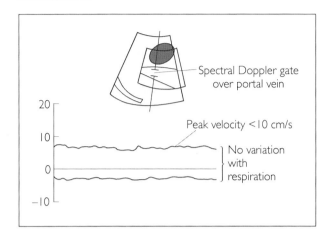

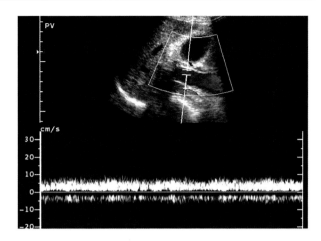

1b Portal hypertension (severe)

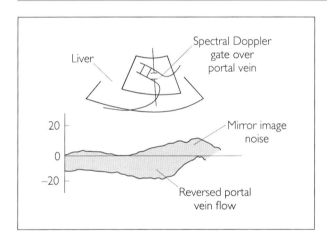

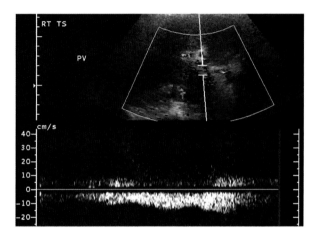

2 Portal vein thrombosis

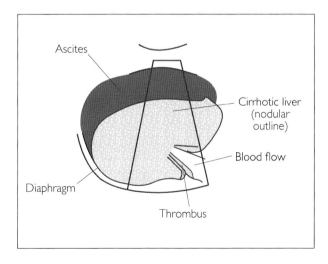

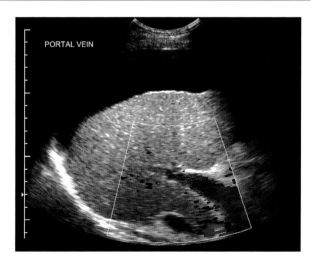

● 3 Budd–Chiari syndrome

This is obstruction of hepatic veins by thrombus, tumour or a congenital fibrous web. The risk factors include pregnancy, malignancy, coagulation disorders and the oral contraceptive pill. In >50% of cases, it is idiopathic. Note that the same features may arise from IVC thrombosis.

Ultrasound features
- Acute stage: hepatomegaly
- Chronic stage: cirrhosis, regenerative nodules, enlargement of caudate lobe
- Splenomegaly
- Ascites
- Colour Doppler:
  - intrahepatic collaterals
  - reversed/no flow in hepatic veins, with or without stenotic segments
  - vein–vein shunting from one vein to another
- Spectral Doppler:
  - loss of normal hepatic vein triphasic waveform
  - waveform may be absent, turbulent, reversed or monophasic
  - reversed flow in IVC

● *Appendix: Explanation of triphasic hepatic vein waveform*

The hepatic vein waveform corresponds to the venous pressure in the right atrium. The pressure from the right atrium is transmitted to the hepatic veins via the IVC.

1 During atrial systole, there is back-pressure to the IVC and hepatic veins. The hepatic flow is towards the probe, i.e. hepatopetal and away from the heart.

2 The tricuspid valve then closes and the right ventricle contracts. During ventricular systole, the right atrium fills passively, and therefore the hepatic flow is towards the heart, i.e. hepatofugal.

3 As the right atrium fills with blood, the pressure increases, resulting in a slower rate of flow into the right atrium.

4 The tricuspid valve opens at the end of ventricular systole, the right atrial pressure drops slightly, and so the rate of flow into the right atrium increases again.

5 Blood passively fills the right ventricle during ventricular diastole, resulting in a pressure rise.

6 At the end of ventricular diastole, the atrium contracts, resulting again in a surge of pressure, which is transmitted to the hepatic vein waveform.

WHAT TO LOOK FOR

SCAN IMAGE

3 Budd–Chiari syndrome

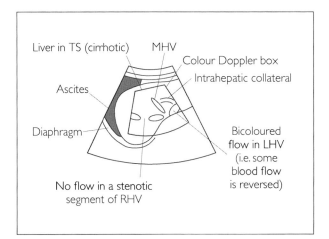

Liver in TS (cirrhotic)   MHV
Colour Doppler box
Intrahepatic collateral
Ascites
Diaphragm
Bicoloured flow in LHV (i.e. some blood flow is reversed)
No flow in a stenotic segment of RHV

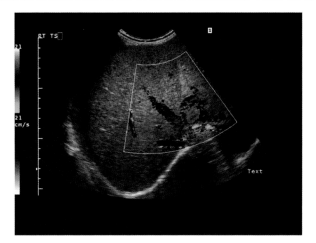

Appendix: Triphasic hepatic vein waveform

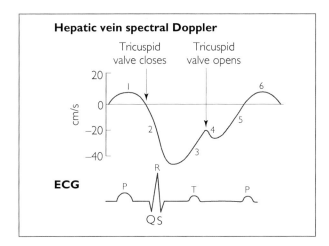

Hepatic vein spectral Doppler

Tricuspid valve closes   Tricuspid valve opens

cm/s

ECG

POST-TRANSPLANT: ANATOMY

The surgical procedure of liver transplantation comprises:

1. A cholecystectomy.
2. An orthotopic transplant (i.e. the transplant liver is in the same anatomical position as the native organ), with five surgical anastomoses:
   (i) suprahepatic IVC
   (ii) infrahepatic IVC
   (iii) main portal vein
   (iv) hepatic artery
   (v) CBD (usually to a Roux bowel loop)

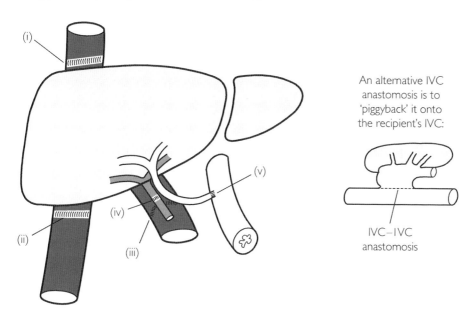

An alternative IVC anastomosis is to 'piggyback' it onto the recipient's IVC:

IVC–IVC anastomosis

POST-TRANSPLANT: MAIN AIMS OF THE SCAN

● *Assess for postoperative complications*
- Anastomotic leaks/hematoma/stenosis/thrombosis
- Bile duct leaks/biloma/stenosis/stricture
- Infection/hepatic abscess

● *Assess for immunosuppression side-effects*
- Undersuppressed: rejection
- Oversuppressed: renal impairment

POST-TRANSPLANT: PERFORMING THE SCAN

- **Patient position:** Supine.
- **Preparation:** None.
- **Probe:** Low-frequency (3–5 MHz) curvilinear with a probe cover (risk of cross-infection).
- **Machine:** Select abdomen preset mode.
- **Method:** Document the date of transplant and number of days postoperation. Read the operation note if it is available. The post-transplant scan follows exactly the same steps as the pre-transplant scan. In both scans, a full abdomen protocol scan is completed and Doppler examinations of hepatic artery, hepatic veins, portal vein, splenic vein and inferior vena cava are performed. However, the likely pathologies are different and these are highlighted below. For further details of each step, refer to the pre-transplant protocol. The salient points are summarized below.

PROBE POSITION

INSTRUCTIONS

I Liver

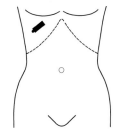

- Place the probe in the RUQ and scan through the liver in TS and LS.
- In a patient who has had a recent transplant, there will be a 'Mercedes sign' surgical scar with dressings and possibly drains. This may interfere with the usual position of the probe for scanning. Therefore try angling the probe around the dressings or using an intercostal approach.
- Examine the liver parenchyma for:
  - any focal lesions
  - areas of infarction (hepatic artery insufficiency)
  - abscess
  - recurrence of HCC
  - PTLD
- Examine the subphrenic and subhepatic spaces, looking specifically for:
  - fluid collections, i.e. hematoma
  - biloma, abscess
  - ascites
  - pleural effusion (especially right)
- Note that there are no ultrasound features of rejection – a liver biopsy is needed for diagnosis.
- Acquire representative image(s).
- Please refer to technique outlined in the pre-transplant section.

| **PROBE POSITION** | **INSTRUCTIONS** |

2 CBD

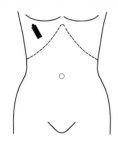

- Examine the CBD in two planes
- Measure its diameter:
  - Dilation can signify cholestasis and ascending infection.
  - Stenosis may signify anastomotic stricture or hepatic artery insufficiency.
- *Hint:* Remember that the gallbladder will have been removed during the transplant operation!
- Acquire representative image(s).

3 MHA spectral Doppler

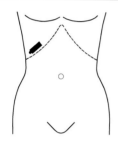

- Adults should be scanned on postoperative day 3. Before this, there may be false positive results due to normal postsurgical features. The local surgical team will have a strong view on the frequency and timing of scans.
- Children should be scanned on postoperative day 1 because they are at a much higher risk of hepatic artery thrombosis.
- Place the probe in the RUQ intercostally. Find the portal vein and then look anterior to it to visualize the main hepatic artery.
- Turn on colour Doppler. Optimize the colour signal and take note of flow in the hepatic artery. Check both the left and right branches.
- If no flow is detected, turn up the colour gain and reduce the PRF. If there is still no flow, try a lower-frequency probe. Consider contrast medium enhancement. If, despite this, no flow is detected, the hepatic artery is likely to be occluded.
- If the flow is detected, turn on spectral Doppler and place the gate over the hepatic artery, acquiring a trace.
- Within 48 hours postoperation, there may just be a small systolic spike with no EDF – this is not significant, and resolves within 48 hours.
- Acquire representative image(s).

4 MPV spectral Doppler

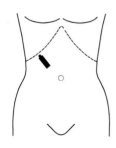

- Find the portal vein by placing the probe perpendicular to the right costal margin MCL.
- Turn on colour Doppler and assess patency.
- Turn on spectral Doppler and place the gate over the portal vein, acquiring a trace.
- Measure the peak velocity.
- Record the direction and character of flow.
- Post-surgery, the waveform usually appears turbulent around the anastomotic site. This is not significant unless it is associated with high peak velocities >100 cm/s.
- Acquire representative image(s).

PROBE POSITION   **INSTRUCTIONS**

5 Hepatic veins spectral Doppler

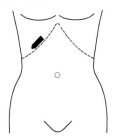

Repeat this step exactly as for the pre-transplant scan. The technique is the same:

- Turn on colour Doppler and assess the patency of all three hepatic veins.
- Turn on spectral Doppler and place the gate over a hepatic vein, acquiring a trace.
- Acquire representative image(s).

6 IVC spectral Doppler

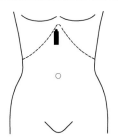

Repeat this step exactly as for the pre-transplant scan. The technique is the same:

- Turn on colour Doppler to assess patency.
- Turn on spectral Doppler and place the gate over the IVC, acquiring a trace.
- Acquire representative image(s).

7 Splenic vein spectral Doppler

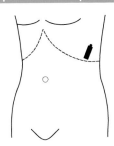

- Ask the patient to turn 45° onto the right side.
- Measure the spleen length. Note that if the spleen was enlarged prior to surgery then it will remain so in the early postoperative phase.
- Turn on colour Doppler and locate the splenic vein. Is the vein patent? Are there any varices? Note that varices may still be present in the initial postoperative phase.
- Turn on spectral Doppler and place the gate over the splenic vein, acquiring a trace.
- Acquire representative image(s).

8 Kidneys

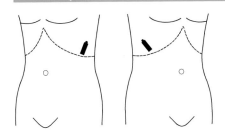

- Scan through both kidneys in two planes as for the abdominal ultrasound protocol.
- Look specifically for any evidence of renal impairment (a side-effect of the immunosuppressive drugs or due to intraoperative hypotension):
  - swollen enlarged kidneys
  - echo-bright cortex
- Acquire representative image(s).

POST-TRANSPLANT: PATHOLOGY

● 1 Post-transplant collection

The main differential is between a hematoma and a biloma:

Hematoma

Most transplants have an immediate postoperative hematoma, usually in the gallbladder fossa. This is usually due to the trauma of surgery. If the patient is asymptomatic, no action is required. Beware of a painful or rapidly enlarging hematoma – this may represent a vascular anastomotic leak and requires further investigation.

Ultrasound features
- In early stages, seen as an echo-free area
- May later contain echo-bright fibrin strands
- Adjacent to the liver and often posterior to the right lobe

Biloma

This is a collection of bile due to a bile duct anastomotic leak. It may lead to peritonitis. Bilomas usually occur in the first 2 months postoperation.

Ultrasound features
- Echo-poor collection
- May have internal echoes if sludge forms
- Occurs adjacent to the bile duct, either intra- or extraheptic

Note that ultrasound cannot differentiate reliably between blood, ascites, bile and pus.

● 2 Bile duct stricture

This occurs in 15% of transplant patients. It may occur many years after transplant. Stricture may be due either to the technical complications of the anastomosis or to diffuse injury secondary to hepatic artery thrombosis, rejection, etc.

Ultrasound features
- Narrowing of CBD
- Proximal intrahepatic duct dilatation

● 3 Post-transplant lymphoproliferative disorder

This occurs in 10% of transplant patients. It is a malignant disease with a proliferation of B cells in lymph nodes and solid organs. There is an increased risk with high-dose immunosuppressive drugs and in patients with EBV. Post-transplant lymphoproliferative disorder (PTLD) usually occurs within 1 year of transplant.

Ultrasound features
- Single or multiple focal echo-poor masses
- Masses may be vascular
- Can occur in the liver allograft, bowel, kidneys, spleen
- Multiple sites of abdominal lymphadenopathy

WHAT TO LOOK FOR   **SCAN IMAGE**

1 Hematoma

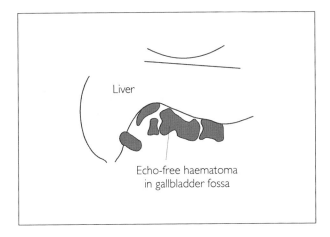

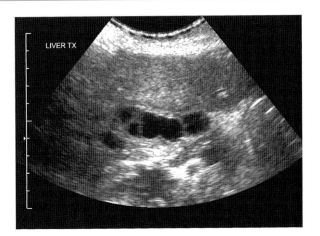

2 CBD stricture

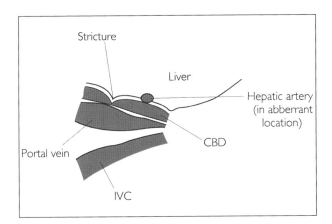

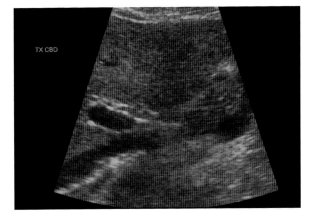

3 PTLD

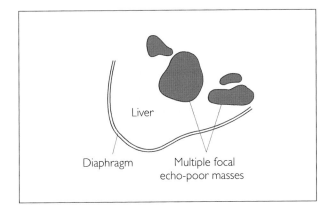

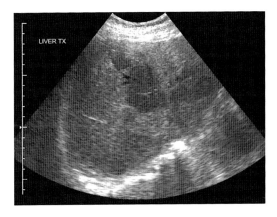

● 4 *Hepatic artery stenosis*

This occurs in approximately 5%–10% of liver transplant patients. It usually occurs within the first few weeks after transplant. Hepatic artery stenosis can lead to hepatic infarction, abscess formation, bile duct necrosis and leakage. If liver abscess can be seen, then there must be hepatic artery stenosis – the hepatic artery is the sole supply to the bile ducts.

Ultrasound features
- arvus tardus' pattern distal to stenosis, i.e. slow systolic upstroke and increased EDF
- Acceleration time >0.08 s
- Resistance index <0.05
- A doubling or more of peak systolic velocity across the stenosis.

If this progresses, it may result in hepatic artery thrombosis.

● 5 *Hepatic artery thrombosis*

This occurs in approximately 5% of liver transplant patients. Complete occlusion of the hepatic artery is a surgical emergency because the artery provides oxygenation for the entire biliary system and therefore the liver quickly infarcts, with consequent biliary stasis, abscess formation and sepsis. The mortality rate without re-transplantation is 75%.

Ultrasound features
- Absent colour Doppler flow
- Absent spectral Doppler waveform
- If collateral flow has developed, it may be seen as a 'parvus tardus' pattern

● 6 *Hepatic vein thrombosis*

Look specifically for hepatic vein thrombosis in patients who have previously had Budd–Chiari syndrome, as they are at increased risk of re-thrombosis.

Ultrasound features
- Expansion of vein: complete/partial loss of colour Doppler signal
- Internal echoes within the vein
- Splenomegaly
- Ascites
- Colour Doppler:
  - intrahepatic collaterals
  - reversed/no flow in hepatic veins, possibly with stenotic segments
  - vein–vein shunting from one vein to another
- Spectral Doppler:
  - loss of normal hepatic vein triphasic waveform
  - waveform may be absent, turbulent, reversed or monophasic
  - reversed flow in IVC

WHAT TO LOOK FOR   **SCAN IMAGE**

4 Hepatic artery stenosis

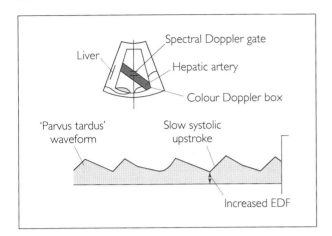

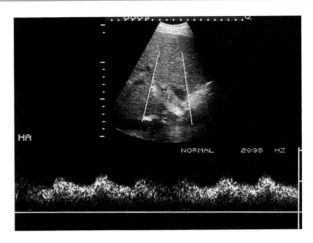

6a Hepatic vein thrombosis spectral Doppler

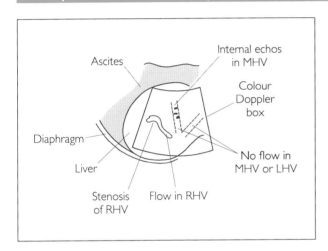

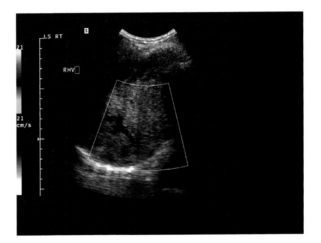

6b Hepatic vein thrombosis colour Doppler

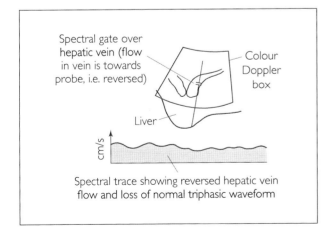

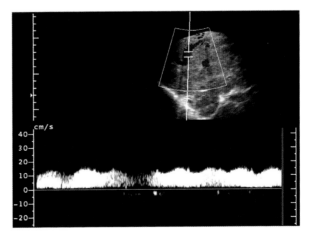

7 Testes

ANATOMY

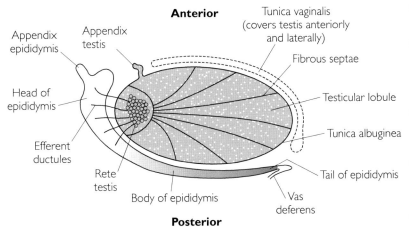

- Normal testes have homogeneous echotexture.
- Fine echo-bright fibrous septae continuous with the tunica albuginea run through the gland, dividing it into lobules.
- Seminiferous tubules in the lobules converge to become larger straight tubules at the rete testis.
- The head of the epididymis contains converging tubules and is of a similar echotexture to the body of the testis.
- The body and tail of the epididymis appear more echo-poor.

(ii) TS: anatomy

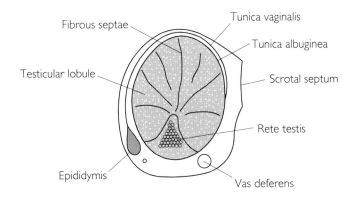

(iv) Venous drainage

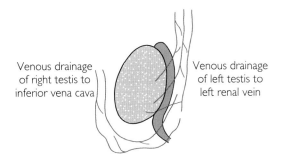

- The pampiniform venous plexus drains the testis.
- The cremasteric plexus drains the epididymis and scrotal wall.
- Both freely anastomose.

(iii) Arterial blood supply

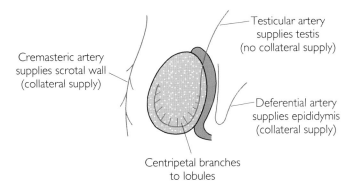

DOI: 10.1201/9781003381655-7

PERFORMING THE SCAN

- **Preparation:** Obtain consent for the examination. A chaperone is advised for all (male and female) examiners.
- **Patient position:** Supine with towel under scrotum to lift it anterior to the upper thighs and aid access. Ask the patient to hold the penis out of the way.
- **Probe:** High-frequency (6–17 MHz) linear.
- **Machine:** Select small-parts/testis preset mode, use multiple focal zones, turn off tissue harmonics, use compound imaging, parallel function and adjust the frequency to optimize images.
- **Method:** Acquire more than just representative images for each step if pathology is found.

PROBE POSITION	INSTRUCTIONS

1 LS: testis

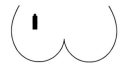

- Begin by placing the probe in the sagittal (LS) plane on the right testis.
- Look for the body of the testis and alter the depth until the epididymis can be seen behind it. Adjust the FOV accordingly.
- Scan through the testis in LS, observing:
  - normal homogeneous echotexture?
  - any masses, cysts or calcifications?
  - any peripheral fluid collections?
- Also observe the epididymis:
  - any swelling or echotexture abnormalities?
  - any cystic areas?
  - any dilated vessels posteriorly?
- Acquire a representative image.

2 TS: testis

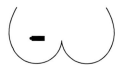

- Turn the probe 90° anticlockwise to scan in TS.
- Scan up and down through the testis and epididymis in this plane, observing for any pathology.
- Acquire a representative image.

3 Testis lateral

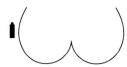

- Place the probe on the lateral aspect of the right testis.
- Scan up and down through the gland in this plane, observing for any pathology as before.
- Acquire a representative image.
- Always remember to ask the patient which bit hurts or to show exactly where any lump is that they have felt.
- Make sure to scan carefully over this area.
- Scanning both testes side by side (TS 'spectacle view') is an effective way of comparing echogenicity, helping detect subtle differences that can point to pathology.

Repeat all of the above on the left side.

WHAT TO LOOK FOR

SCAN IMAGE

1

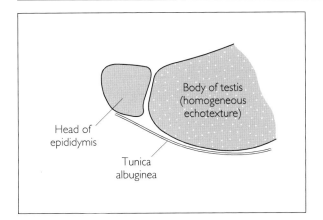

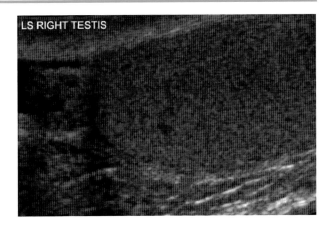

2

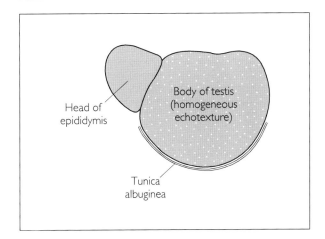

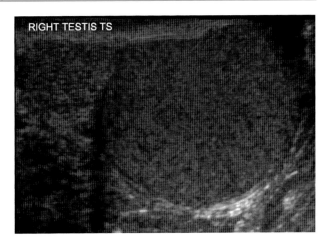

3

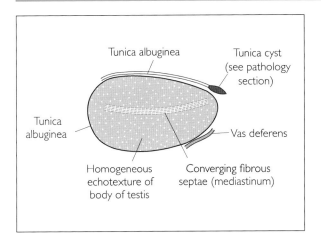

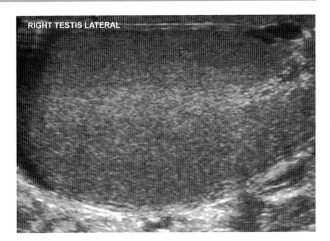

● *Suspected varicocele*

- Look for tortuous, dilated (>2 mm) veins posterior to the epididymis. *Hint:* 90% occur on the left side.
- Colour or power Doppler will demonstrate strong blood flow within them.
- Scanning as the patient strains or stands up should demonstrate that the vessels increase in size. Young men do not need the kidneys and renal veins checking. However, older men with a recently acquired varicocele should have these checked. There is a small risk of renal carcinoma being the underlying cause.
- See the pathology section for more on this condition.

● *The painful testis (suspected torsion/ epididymo-orchitis)*

- Use power Doppler to compare blood flow in both testes.
- Optimize the Doppler signal: Adjust the colour gain and focus position, magnify the image, reduce the colour box size, and set the filter and PRF at low.
- Look for normal perfusion, which should be out to the edges.
- If the painful testis has increased blood flow, this *may* be an orchitis.
- If the painful testis has reduced blood flow, this *may* be a torsion.
- See the pathology section for more on these conditions.

● *Infertility referral*

- It is necessary to measure the testicular volumes (normal >10 cm^3).
- Calculate from LS and TS images, measuring the diameter in three planes.
- The split-screen function can be helpful for this.
- Use the measurement package to calculate the volume (on most machines).
- Remember to also examine carefully for secondary causes of subfertility, such as tumours and varicoceles.

WHAT TO LOOK FOR

SCAN IMAGE

● *Suspected varicocele*

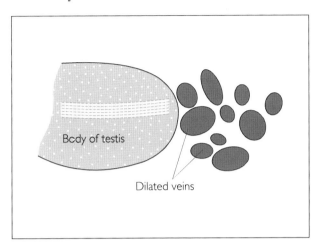

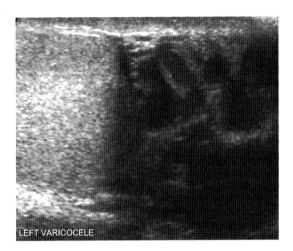

● *Painful testis*

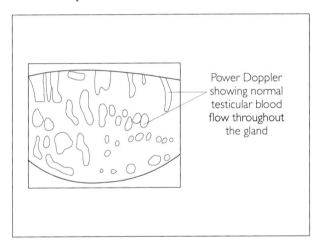

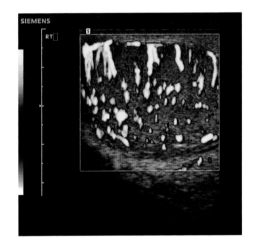

● *Infertility referral*

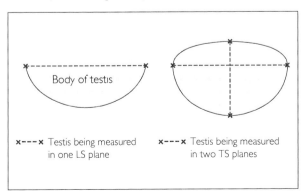

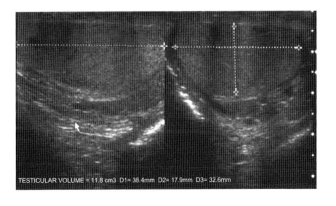

TESTES: PATHOLOGY

● 1 Benign cystic lesions

(a) Intratesticular cyst
This is usually an incidental finding. Intratesticular cysts are located within the body of the testis and display typical features of a simple cyst:
- smooth edge
- thin wall
- echo-free contents
- postacoustic enhancement

(b) Epididymal cyst
This is a very common finding (up to 40% of men). It may present clinically as a smooth firm lump above the testis (caused by outpouchings of the epididymal tubules).

Ultrasound features
- Most commonly located in the epididymal head
- Displays the typical features of a simple cyst

(c) Tunica albuginea cyst
This presents clinically as a testicular lump, mimicking a tumour. This lesion is commonly discovered on self-examination, as it distorts the smooth testicular contour.

Ultrasound features
- Located on the periphery of the body of the testis (paratesticular)
- Displays the typical features of a simple cyst

WHAT TO LOOK FOR　　　　　　　　**SCAN IMAGE**

1a Intratesticular cyst

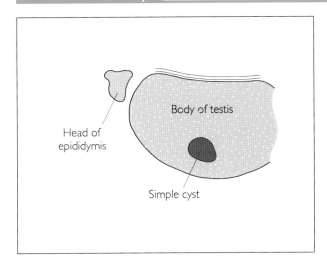

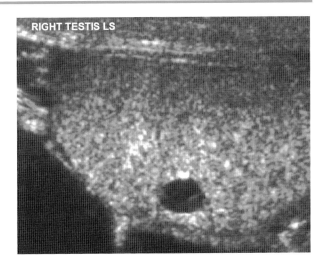

1b Epididymal cyst

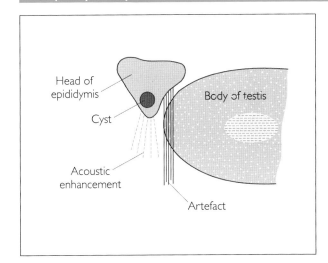

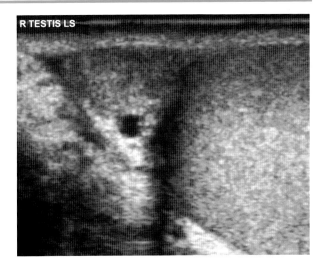

1c Tunica albuginea cyst

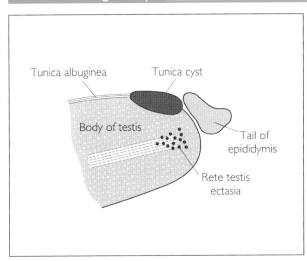

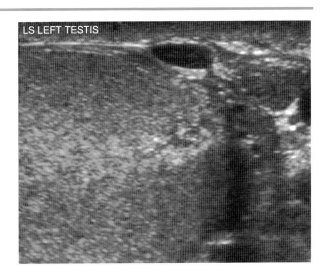

● 2 Hydrocele

This is fluid accumulation between the two layers of the tunica vaginalis. It can be:
- Congenital: due to non-closure of the processus vaginalis
- Acquired: trauma, tumour, inflammation (these may contain debris)

Ultrasound features
- Seen as an echo-free area typically surrounding the anterolateral aspect of the testis.
- Occasionally, fine septations or echo-bright debris may be seen within the fluid

● 3 Varicoceles

These are dilations of the papiniform veins that drain the testis and are caused by incompetent vein valves. They are common (around 10% of males in their teens and twenties), with 90% occurring on the left side. Clinically, they may cause a dull scrotal ache and soft scrotal swelling. They can be associated with a low sperm count.

Ultrasound features
- Seen as tortuous dilated (>2mm) echo-free structures
- Located posterior to the epididymis
- The vessels increase in size on straining or standing upright
- The vessels show strong blood flow on colour or power Doppler

Rarely, a varicocele is due to a renal tumour obstructing venous return from the testicular veins. It is therefore important to image the kidneys as well in older men with a new varicocele.

● 4 Postvasectomy changes

These are thought to be caused by a combination of back-pressure effects and low-grade inflammatory reaction. They are usually bilateral and asymptomatic.

Ultrasound features
- The epididymis appears thickened (>3mm) and echo-poor, with multiple small punctate cystic areas

WHAT TO LOOK FOR   **SCAN IMAGE**

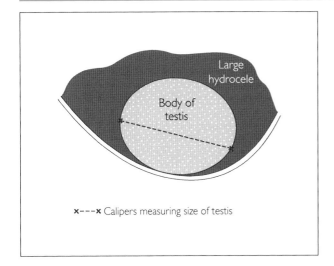

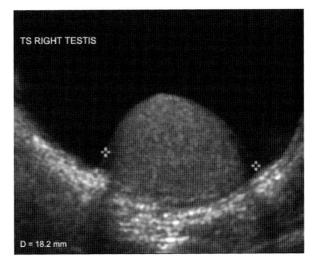

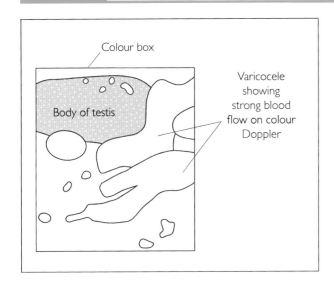

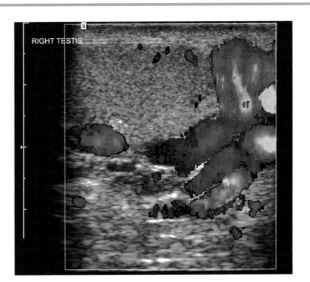

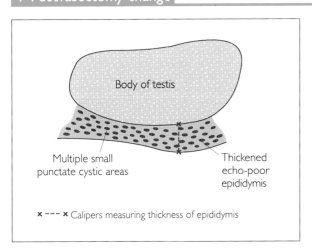

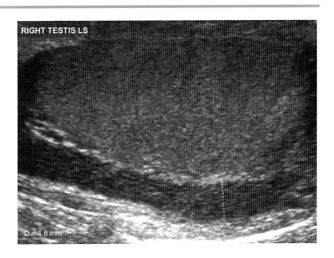

● 5 Testicular microlithiasis

These multiple small calcific foci are usually an incidental finding, but some studies have shown an increased risk of developing a testicular malignancy and subfertility.

Ultrasound features

- More than five echo-bright foci (each <3 mm) within the body of the testis

Hint: Patients with microlithoasis are advised to perform regular self-examination, and if any new lumps are detected a repeat ultrasound should be performed.

● 6 Testicular tumours

As a rule, most intratesticular masses are malignant. The most common tumour type is the seminoma.

Ultrasound features

- Variable appearances: tumours can appear as echo-poor, cystic or mixed echogenicity masses.

Note: A urologist should be contacted immediately with the result if a tumour is found. Consider checking the para-aortic region for nodal spread.

WHAT TO LOOK FOR

SCAN IMAGE

5 Testicular microlithiasis

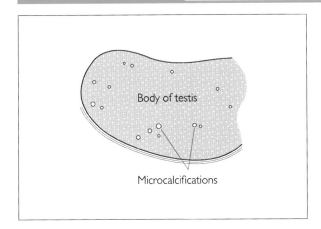

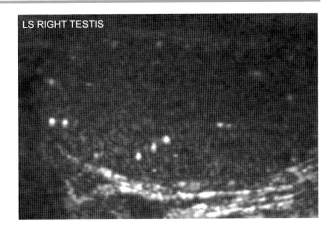

LS RIGHT TESTIS

6a Testicular tumour

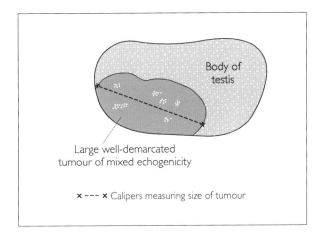

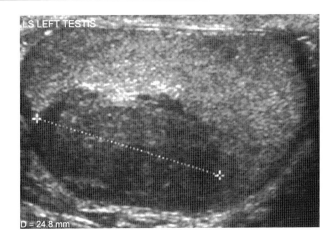

LS LEFT TESTIS

D = 24.8 mm

● 7 *Epididymo-orchitis*

This is caused by ascending spread of infection (e.g. chlamydia, gonorrhoea) or by the blood-borne route (e.g. mumps). It is commonly seen in young males. The majority of cases are unilateral and of epididymitis only.

Ultrasound features
- Epididymis appears swollen (>3 mm) and of mixed echogenicity; the tail is the most common part affected
- Colour/power Doppler flow is increased over the affected area in the acute phase
- There may be a reactive hydrocele
- Oedematous thickening of overlying scrotal skin is common
- Rarely, the condition can progress to abscess formation
- If the testis is involved, this appears swollen, with echo-poor areas (uniform or focal)
- Colour/power Doppler flow in the testes is increased, but in very severe cases it may be reduced, causing diagnostic confusion with testicular torsion

● 8 *Testicular torsion*

This is twisting of the spermatic cord resulting in testicular ischaemia. It is usually caused by the 'bell-clapper' anatomical variant, in which the tunica vaginalis extends around posterior to the testis, allowing it to twist more easily. Torsion can be complete (360° twist), partial or intermittent (torsion/detorsion).

Ultrasound features
- Testis appears echo-poor; it often has a reactive hydrocele
- The hallmark is reduced/absent intratesticular blood flow using power Doppler (see earlier). Note that the epididymis may show increased flow, as it has a collateral blood supply

Note:
- Beware false-positives: severe epididymo-orchitis
- Beware false-negatives: intermittent torsion/detorsion

Torsion is an emergency requiring prompt surgical intervention to prevent testicular infarction. Many consider that ultrasound should not be used for diagnosis as it may delay time to surgery and there is also a risk of a false negative appearance with the torsion/detorsion sequence.

WHAT TO LOOK FOR   SCAN IMAGE

7 Epididymo-orchitis

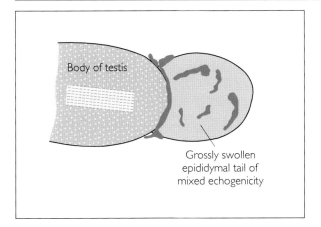

Body of testis

Grossly swollen
epididymal tail of
mixed echogenicity

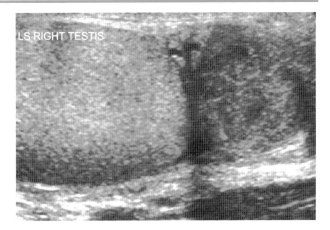

LS RIGHT TESTIS

8 Testicular infarction

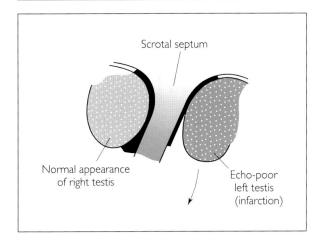

Scrotal septum

Normal appearance
of right testis

Echo-poor
left testis
(infarction)

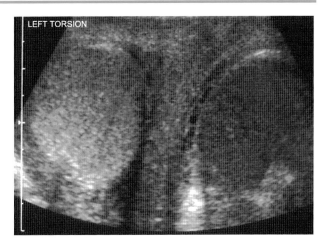

LEFT TORSION

● 9 *Torsion of testicular appendix*

Presents with sudden onset of scrotal pain and swelling; this can mimic testicular torsion. However, the condition requires no surgical intervention and resolves spontaneously. The appendix will often detach itself and come to lie free within the scrotal sac, where it may calcify to become a scrotolith (scrotal pearl).

Ultrasound features
● Acutely, the appendix appears enlarged due to oedema, often with a reactive hydrocele
● A scrotolith is a small mobile echo-bright structure within the scrotal sac

WHAT TO LOOK FOR

SCAN IMAGE

9 Past torsion of testicular appendix

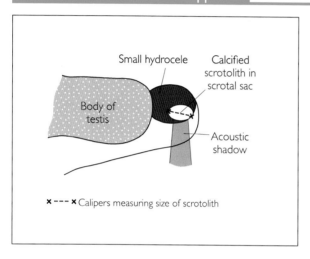

Small hydrocele Calcified scrotolith in scrotal sac

Body of testis

Acoustic shadow

x---x Calipers measuring size of scrotolith

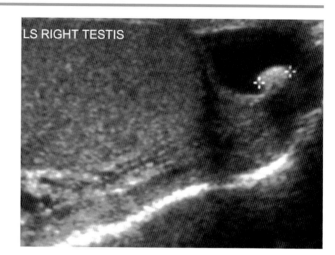

LS RIGHT TESTIS

8 *Lower limb veins*

ANATOMY

Deep veins of right leg

Superficial veins of right leg

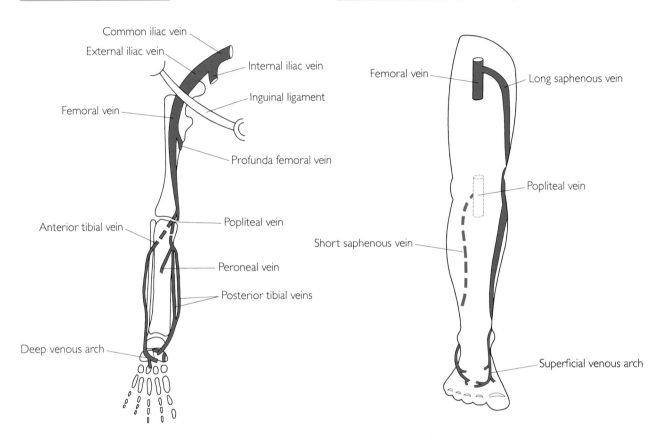

● *Key points*

1 The superficial veins drain into the deep veins.
2 The deep veins and perforating veins contain valves.
3 25% of people have duplicated femoral or popliteal veins – always scan both vessel lumens (3% have triple femoral or popliteal veins).
4 The femoral vein is *deep* to the femoral artery.
5 The popliteal vein is *superficial* to the popliteal artery.

DOI: 10.1201/9781003381655-8

PERFORMING THE SCAN

- **Patient position:** Sit up with leg exposed from groin to toes. Sitting up helps to distend the leg veins and make them easier to scan.
- **Preparation:** Nil.
- **Probe:** High-frequency (5–8 MHz) linear (for a very obese/swollen leg, consider using a low-frequency (3–5 MHz) curvilinear probe).
- **Machine:** Select the venous vascular preset mode. Use tissue harmonics if the SNR is poor. Use a dual screen when acquiring images with and without compression in TS.
- **Method:** Start at the groin and scan distally. If a thrombus is found:
  - (a) STOP scanning distally, as there is a risk of dislodging the thrombus.
  - (b) Scan proximally to examine the extent of the thrombus, i.e. if there is femoral vein DVT, scan the iliac vein; if there is iliac vein DVT, scan the IVC, etc.
  - (c) Use colour Doppler to distinguish occlusive versus non-occlusive thrombus.

  Always scan the bit that the patient says hurts.

PROBE POSITION	INSTRUCTIONS

1 TS: proximal femoral vein

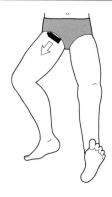

- Sit patient up to increase venous dilation. The patient bends the knee and externally rotates the hip so that the leg falls out laterally.
- Place the probe in the groin crease to find the proximal femoral vein in TS. Adjust the focus to the level of the vessel.
- Look for the 'Mickey Mouse sign' – the head of Mickey is the femoral vein, and the ears are the femoral artery (laterally) and the long saphenous vein (medially).
- Compress the vein with the probe. Push gently along the axis of the probe with the probe held perpendicular to the skin and compressing the vein against the underlying bone:
  - complete compression of the vein = no thrombus
  - partial or no compression = thrombus
- Acquire one image without compression and one image with compression.

2 TS: mid femoral vein

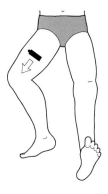

- Keep scanning in TS.
- Follow the femoral vein down to mid-thigh.
- Compress intermittently, i.e. every 1 cm:
  - complete compression of the vein = no thrombus
  - partial or no compression = thrombus
- Increase the depth on descending the leg.
- Keep the focus on the level of the vessel.
- Use colour Doppler to aid in locating the vein.
- Acquire one image without compression and one image with compression.

WHAT TO LOOK FOR

SCAN IMAGE

1 (Dual screen)

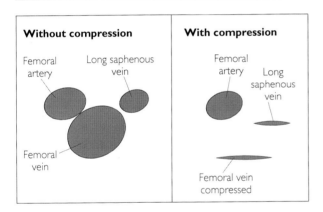

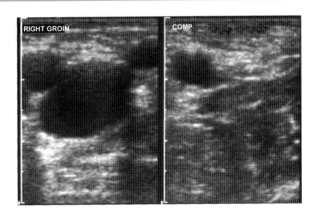

2

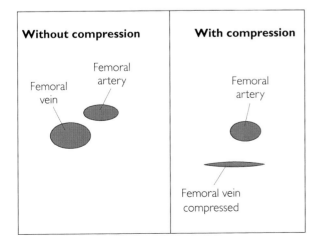

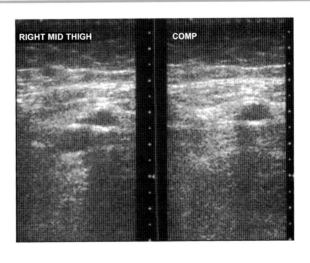

PROBE POSITION   **INSTRUCTIONS**

3 TS: distal femoral vein

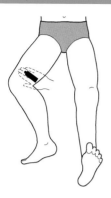

- Keep scanning in TS.
- Follow the course of the femoral vein down to the knee, and continue to compress intermittently.
- At the lower one-third of the thigh, the femoral vein enters the adductor canal, and it becomes more difficult to compress the vein against the femur. Therefore, try putting the free hand under the leg and pushing up against the probe to test for full compression.
- Acquire one image without compression and one image with compression.

4 LS: femoral vein

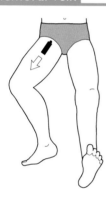

- Now scan the femoral vein in LS.
- Go back to the groin and find the femoral vein first in TS; then rotate the probe through 90° clockwise to scan in LS.
- Follow the femoral vein down to the knee. Look for small non-occlusive thrombi in the vessel wall, especially around the valves.
- Turn on colour Doppler and set the PRF, colour gain, wall filter, etc. to optimize edge definition and avoid colour flow bleeding out of the vein.
- Scan the femoral vein again in LS with colour, looking for filling defects, i.e. non-occlusive thrombi. Measure any abnormalities seen (size of thrombus, lymph nodes, etc.).
- Acquire one or two representative images.

5 TS: popliteal vein

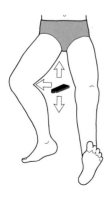

- Now scan the popliteal vein in TS.
- Place the probe in the popliteal fossa and look for the popliteal vein (more superficial than the artery).
- Push the probe against the posterior tibia to check for complete compression.
- Acquire one image without compression and one image with compression.

WHAT TO LOOK FOR

SCAN IMAGE

3 (Dual screen)

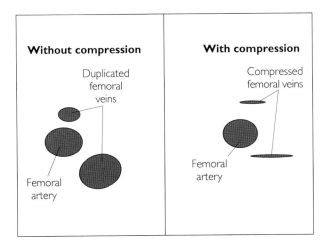

Without compression

Duplicated femoral veins

Femoral artery

With compression

Compressed femoral veins

Femoral artery

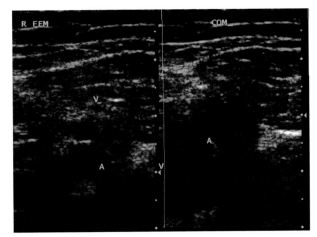

4

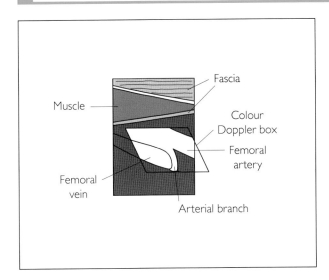

Muscle

Fascia

Colour Doppler box

Femoral artery

Femoral vein

Arterial branch

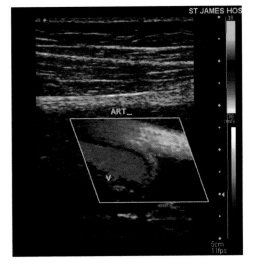

5 (Dual screen)

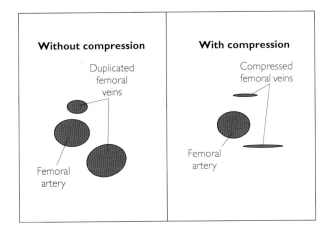

Without compression

Duplicated femoral veins

Femoral artery

With compression

Compressed femoral veins

Femoral artery

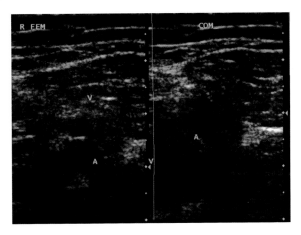

PROBE POSITION   **INSTRUCTIONS**

6 LS: popliteal vein

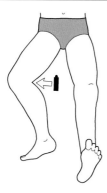

- Now scan the popliteal vein(s) in LS. To do this, find the popliteal vein in TS and then rotate the probe through 90° clockwise.
- Look for small non-occlusive thrombi on the vessel wall.
- Turn on colour Doppler and scan the popliteal vein again in LS, looking for filling defects, i.e. non-occlusive thrombi.
- Measure any abnormalities seen.
- Acquire representative image(s).

7 LS: posterior tibial veins

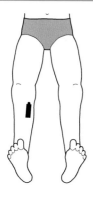

- Now scan the posterior tibial veins.
- Place the probe medial to the mid tibia.
- Look for three calf vessels: two posterior tibial veins laterally and one posterior tibial artery in between. It is easiest to start mid-tibia and then scan up and down the vessels. The veins are often difficult to visualize without colour Doppler.
- Put colour on (there is usually very little flow). To check for patency, squeeze the ankle and look for increased flow in the veins.
- Acquire one image without ankle squeezing and one image with squeezing.
- The peroneal and anterior tibial veins are less likely to have isolated thrombus and so are not routinely included in our protocol. However, it is vital to scan the area the patient has symptoms. It may show thrombus in these veins or it may find superficial thrombophlebitis or muscle tears as a differential diagnosis.

WHAT TO LOOK FOR   **SCAN IMAGE**

6

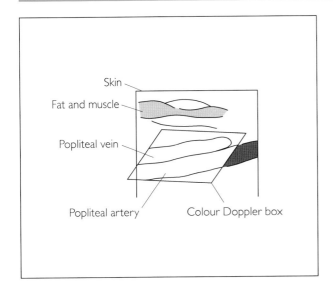

Skin
Fat and muscle
Popliteal vein
Popliteal artery   Colour Doppler box

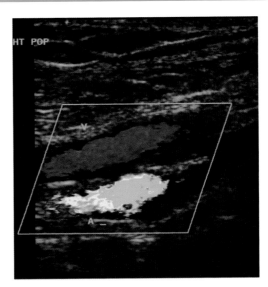

7

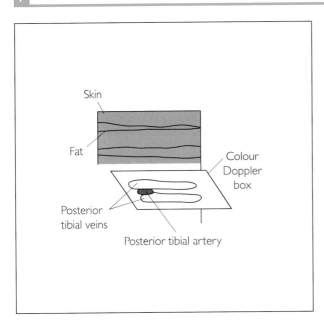

Skin
Fat
Colour
Doppler
box
Posterior tibial veins
Posterior tibial artery

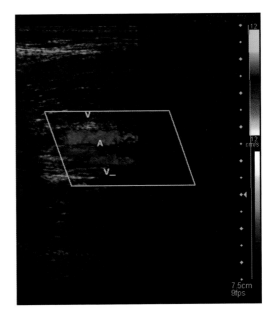

LOWER LIMBS: COMMON PATHOLOGY

● 1 *Deep vein thrombosis*

Risk factors include age, immobility, IVDU, malignancy, obesity, OCP, pregnancy and surgery. DVT presents as a painful swollen limb. The differential diagnosis includes cellulitis, ruptured Baker's cyst and hematoma.

The scan should be repeated after 1 week if symptoms/signs of a thrombosis persist despite a normal scan.

Ultrasound features

- Acute (<1 week): echo-free thrombus in a swollen vein
- Chronic: echo-bright thrombus in a contracted vein, sometimes with tortuous recanalization

	Occlusion due to thrombosis	Stenosis due to thrombosis
TS with compression	Non-compressible	Incompletely compressible
LS with colour Doppler	No flow	Filling defect
LS with spectral Doppler	No flow	Increased velocity at stenosis

Below-knee DVT

- This is a DVT confined to the deep calf veins
- Normal calf veins often have undetectable colour flow so the absence of colour flow alone does not establish the diagnosis
- An expanded vein that does not demonstrate flow with manual ankle compression suggests the diagnosis
- Isolated below-knee DVT is not associated with pulmonary embolism
- Without treatment approximately 20% propagate into the popliteal veins with the potential to embolize to the lungs; serial scans are therefore required to monitor for progression/resolution

WHAT TO LOOK FOR

SCAN IMAGE

1a DVT in TS (Dual screen)

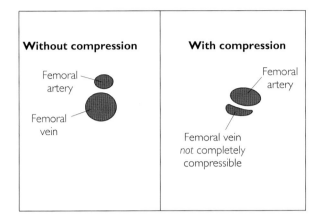

Without compression

Femoral artery

Femoral vein

With compression

Femoral artery

Femoral vein *not* completely compressible

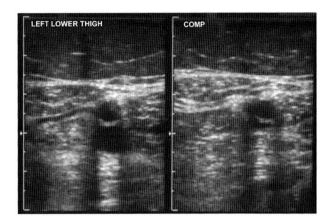

1b DVT in LS

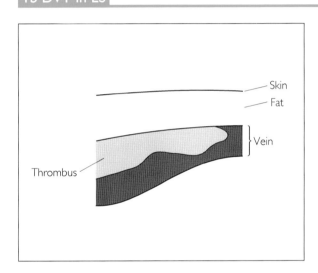

Skin

Fat

Vein

Thrombus

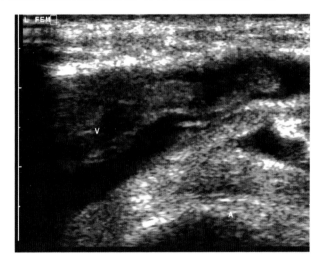

1c DVT with colour Doppler

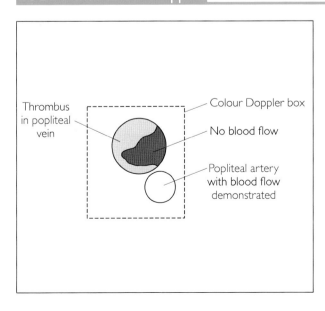

Thrombus in popliteal vein

Colour Doppler box

No blood flow

Popliteal artery with blood flow demonstrated

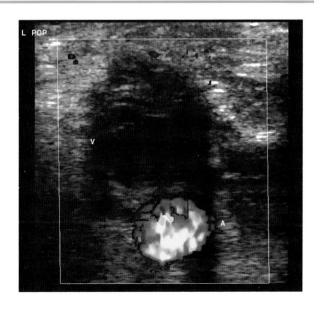

● 2 Baker's cyst

Baker's cysts arise between the medial head of the gastrocnemius and the semimembranosus tendons. They cause pain and swelling when they rupture.

Ultrasound features
- Found on the medial side of the popliteal fossa
- Oval/crescent shape
- Usually echo-free
- Communicates with the knee joint and appears as a 'speech bubble' sign
- When the cyst ruptures, it may extend into the calf, causing swelling

● 3 Hematoma

This can mimic a DVT (i.e. pain and limb swelling). It is usually due to a muscle tear or external trauma.

Ultrasound features
- Within soft tissues/muscles
- Well-defined margins
- Predominantly echo-poor; may contain echo-bright fibrin strands

● 4 Cellulitis

This is infection of the subcutaneous tissues. It presents with a hot, painful, swollen and red limb (or any affected area of the body).

Ultrasound features
- Oedema: fluid between subcutaneous fat, resulting in a 'crazy-paving' effect
- Hyperaemic flow in the vessels

WHAT TO LOOK FOR   SCAN IMAGE

2 Baker's cyst

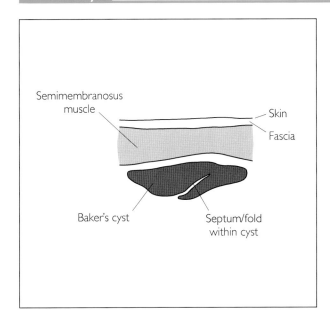

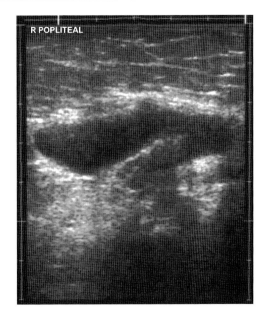

3 Hematoma

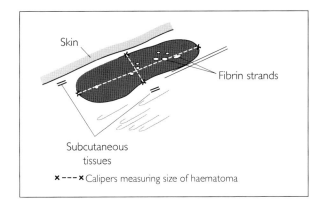

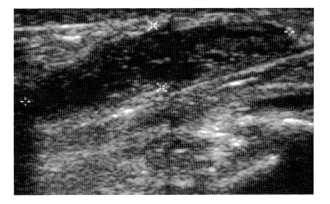

4 Cellulitis

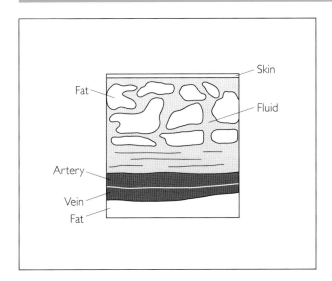

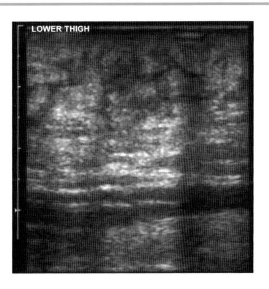

● 5 Thrombophlebitis

This is inflammation, possibly with thrombosis, of the superficial veins, e.g. LSV and SSV.

Ultrasound features
- Superficial vessel wall is irregular/ragged
- Vessel is still compressible

Hint: Check that the thrombus does not extend to the deep system veins.

● 6 Varicose veins

These are dilated tortuous superficial veins. Risk factors include age, pregnancy, family history and obesity.

Ultrasound features
- Dilated tortuous superficial veins

● 7 Lymphadenopathy

Common causes include infection (local or systemic), metastases and lymphoma. It may increase suspicion of cellulitis versus DVT (but keep in mind that the two can coexist!).

Ultrasound features of a normal lymph node
- Elliptical
- Long axis < 10 mm, short axis < 7 mm
- Echo-bright hilum of fat
- Echo-poor cortex

Ultrasound features of an abnormal lymph node
- Spherical
- Long axis > 10 mm
- Loss of echo-bright hilum
- May exert mass effect on surrounding structures

WHAT TO LOOK FOR **SCAN IMAGE**

5 Thrombophlebitis

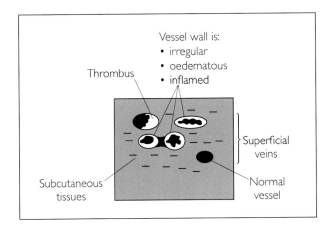

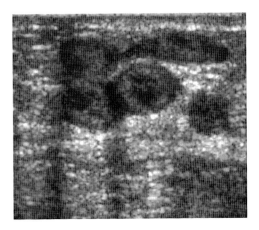

6 Varicose vein

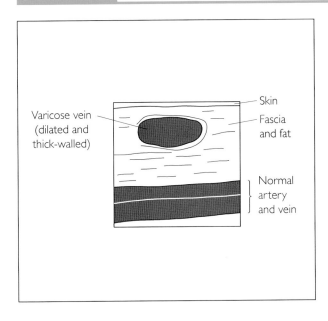

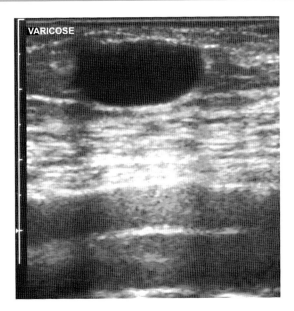

7 Lymph node

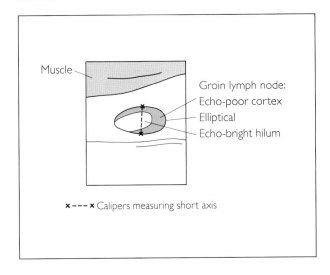

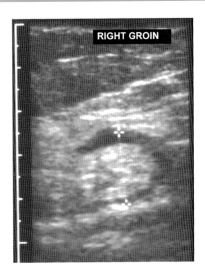

9 Carotid Doppler

ANATOMY

The great vessels

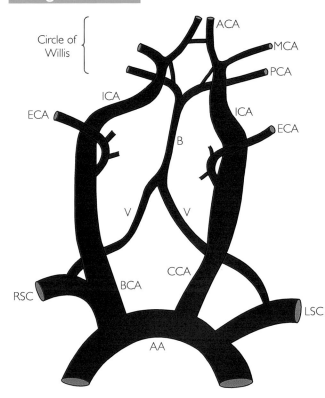

AA   aortic arch
ACA   anterior cerebral artery
B   basilar artery
BCA   brachiocephalic artery
CCA   common carotid artery
ECA   external carotid artery
ICA   internal carotid artery
LSC   left subclavian artery
MCA   middle cerebral artery
PCA   posterior cerebral artery
RSC   right subclavian artery
V   vertebral artery

● Key points

1 The ICA has no branches extracranially.
2 One vertebral artery tends to be more dominant than the other: usually left > right.
3 If the ICA is occluded, there are two collateral pathways:
   (i) the circle of Willis
   (ii) the ophthalmic artery

DOI: 10.1201/9781003381655-9

PERFORMING THE SCAN

- **Patient position:** Neck extended with head turned to the contralateral side.
- **Preparation:** Nil.
- **Probe:** High-frequency (7.5 MHz) linear.
- **Machine:** Select arterial vascular preset mode. Use tissue harmonics and compound imaging. Set the focal zone to the posterior wall of the vessel.
- **Method:** Do not apply any pressure with the probe. Start at the root of the neck and scan cranially along the course of the vessels. Scan both sides of the neck.

PROBE POSITION

INSTRUCTIONS

1 TS: common carotid artery

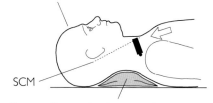

Neck extended and head turned to contralateral side

SCM

Place a pillow under the patient's neck to achieve optimal position

- Begin by placing the probe in TS over the root of the neck, i.e. at the CCA origin.
- Use the SCM as a window to scan through. If the vessel image is not clear, try scanning anterior or posterior to the SCM instead.
- Follow the course of the carotid arteries up the neck as high as possible.
- Look for:
  - level of CCA bifurcation
  - evidence of arterial disease
- Measure any abnormalities seen.
- Acquire representative image(s).

2 LS: carotid arteries

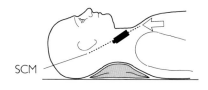

SCM

- Now scan the carotid arteries in LS. To do this, first scan the CCA origin in TS as in Step 1 and then rotate the probe through 90° clockwise so that the CCA is now imaged in LS.
- Follow the course of the carotid arteries up the neck as high as possible.
- The ICA and ECA are in different planes: therefore find the CCA bifurcation, keep the lower portion of the probe over the CCA and rotate the upper portion through small angles to image the ICA and then the ECA separately.
- Look for:
  - atheromatous plaques
  - intima–media thickening (below the CCA bulb, it should be <0.8 mm).
- Acquire representative image(s).

WHAT TO LOOK FOR

SCAN IMAGE

1

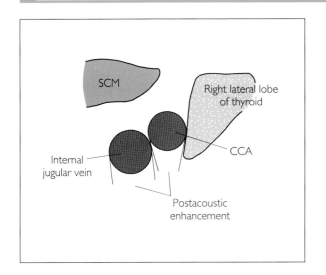

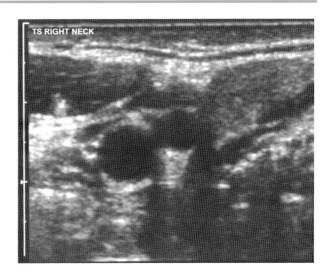

2

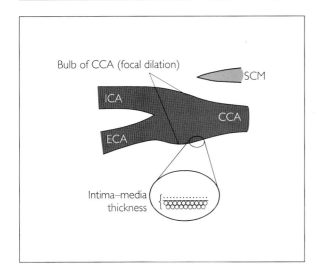

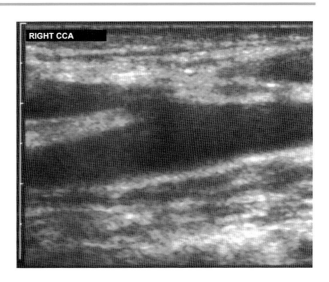

PROBE POSITION	**INSTRUCTIONS**

3 LS: colour Doppler carotid arteries

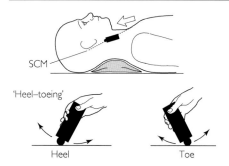

SCM

'Heel–toeing'

Heel   Toe

- Keep scanning the carotids in LS. Turn on colour Doppler and place the colour box over the vessel. Steer the box so that the angle of the box is in the same direction as the vessel flow. 'Heel–toeing' the probe may help get a good angle of Doppler resonation.
- Optimize the colour signal: adjust the colour gain and focus position, narrow the FOV and reduce the colour box size. Set the PRF so that colour aliasing occurs mid-vessel during peak systole.
- Follow the course of the CCA, ICA and ECA up the neck in LS.
- Look for:
    - small branches to identify the ECA
    - velocity change/colour aliasing (stenosis)
    - filling defects (atheromatous plaques)
    - absence of flow (occlusion)
- Acquire representative image(s).

4 LS: spectral Doppler CCA

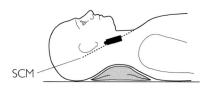

SCM

- Keep scanning in LS with colour Doppler. Select a segment of the CCA. If a stenosis has already been demonstrated, select this segment.
- Now turn on spectral Doppler and place the gate over the CCA at the point of maximum peak velocity, acquiring a trace. Optimize the waveform by adjusting the gate size and ensuring a beam-vessel angle of 40°–60°.
- Select 'calculations' on the machine and then measure the peak velocity. (If no flow is detected with colour Doppler, increase the colour gain and reduce the PRF to increase the sensitivity. If there is still no flow detected, the vessel is occluded.)
- Acquire one or two spectral waveforms. *Hint:* Remember to steer the colour box so that its angle is in the same direction as the vessel flow.

5 LS: spectral Doppler ECA

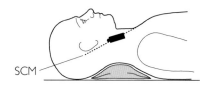

SCM

- Repeat Step 4 for the ECA.
- The normal ECA waveform is:
    - pulsatile with a characteristic notch
    - high resistance flow
    - low diastolic flow
- Acquire one or two spectral waveforms.

Hint: To help identify the ECA versus the ICA, remember that the ECA:

- has extracranial branches – use colour Doppler to help identify them
- demonstrates the 'temporal tapping' phenomena – tap the temporal artery in front of the ear and look for alteration in the spectral waveform of the ECA (there is no effect on the ICA waveform)

WHAT TO LOOK FOR

SCAN IMAGE

3

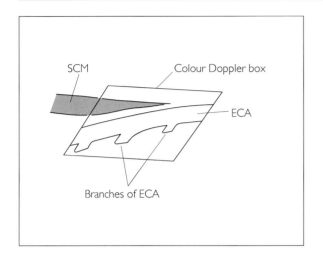

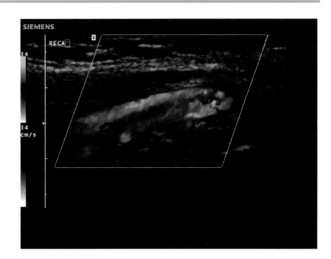

4

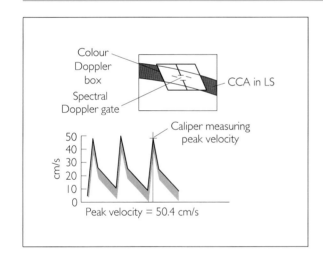

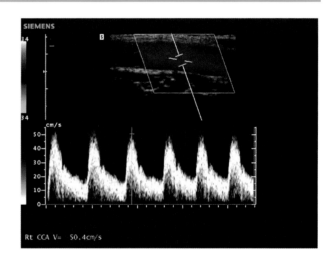

5

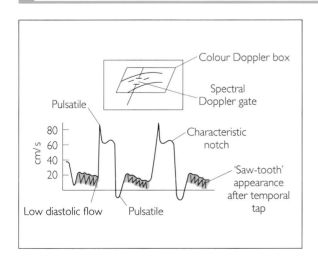

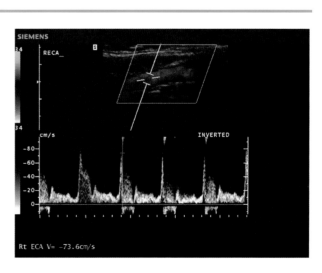

PROBE POSITION	**INSTRUCTIONS**

6 LS: spectral Doppler ICA

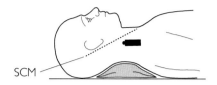

SCM

- Repeat Step 4 for the ICA.
- Measure peak velocity.
- The normal ICA waveform is:
  - less pulsatile than the ECA
  - low resistance flow
  - higher diastolic flow
  - The waveform alone is not reliable in distinguishing the ECA and ICA.
- Acquire one or two spectral waveforms.

Hint: Ensure the beam to flow angle is 40°–60° for accurate velocity measurements.

7 LS: colour Doppler vertebral artery

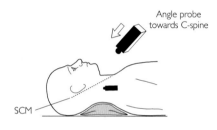

Angle probe towards C-spine

SCM

- Now scan the vertebral artery in LS. Turn off spectral Doppler and keep only colour Doppler switched on.
- To locate the vertebral artery:
  - First find the mid CCA in LS
  - Then angle the probe posteriorly in the direction of the cervical spine
  - Increase the depth and deepen the focus position
  - Look for the vertebral processes (bright echoes) – the vertebral artery and vein lie between them and appear as 'flashes' of colour
- Acquire a representative image.

8 LS: spectral Doppler vertebral artery

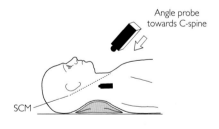

Angle probe towards C-spine

SCM

- Now turn on spectral Doppler and place the gate over the vessel to acquire a spectral waveform as described in Step 4.
- Record the direction of flow only.
- Acquire one or two spectral waveforms.

9 Contralateral-side neck vessels

- Repeat Steps 1–7 for the vessels on the opposite side of the neck.

Do not stand the patient up straightaway at the end of the examination, as they are at risk of a vasovagal episode.

WHAT TO LOOK FOR

SCAN IMAGE

6

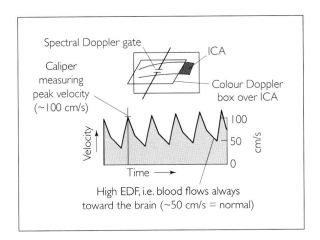

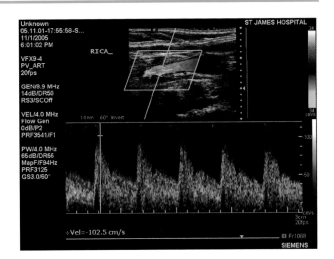

7

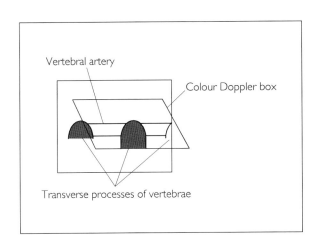

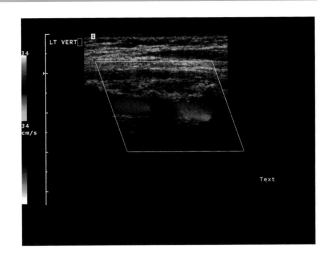

8

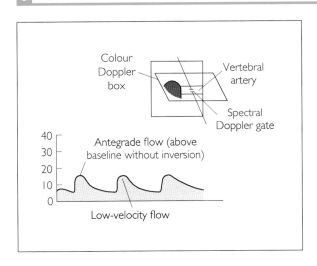

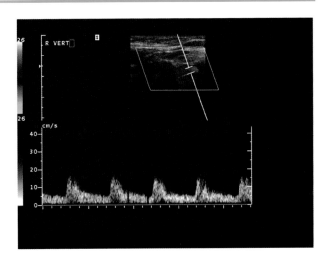

PATHOLOGY

● 1 Atheromatous plaques

Atherosclerosis is a disease of large- and medium-sized muscular arteries. It is characterized by the accumulation of lipids, calcium and cellular debris within the intima of the vessel wall, forming atheromatous plaques. The major risk factors are smoking, hypercholesterolaemia, diabetes and hypertension.

Ultrasound features

- Localized irregular thickening of the vessel wall (measured in TS and LS) causing stenosis
- The echogenicity of the plaque depends on its contents:
  - echo-poor: blood- or lipid-filled = increased risk of rupture
  - echo-bright: calcified = more benign

There are five types of atheromatous plaques, graded according to their ultrasound appearance as below (AC Grey Weale et al. *J Cardiovasc Surg* 1988; 29: 676–81):

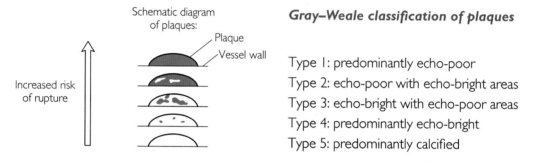

Schematic diagram of plaques:

Plaque
Vessel wall

Increased risk of rupture

Gray–Weale classification of plaques

Type 1: predominantly echo-poor

Type 2: echo-poor with echo-bright areas

Type 3: echo-bright with echo-poor areas

Type 4: predominantly echo-bright

Type 5: predominantly calcified

Across stenosis, there is spectral broadening of the waveform, representing turbulent blood flow and the peak velocity of the blood increases in proportion to the degree of stenosis. Therefore, the degree of stenosis can be estimated by using spectral Doppler to measure the peak velocity.

There are different peak-systolic velocity cut-off values to determine ICA stenosis and the following values are used in Leeds Teaching Hospitals NHS Trust (see Table below). However, it is recommended that you use the agreed cut-off values in your radiology department as there is considerable variation between hospitals.

Peak-systolic velocity (m/s)	Degree of stenosis (%)	Management
<1.5	0–49	Medical
1.5–2.3	50–69	Medical
>2.3	>70	Surgical
None	Occluded	Medical

WHAT TO LOOK FOR　　　　　　　**SCAN IMAGE**

1a Intimal thickening

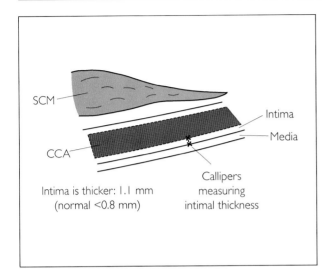

SCM

Intima

Media

CCA

Callipers measuring intimal thickness

Intima is thicker: 1.1 mm (normal <0.8 mm)

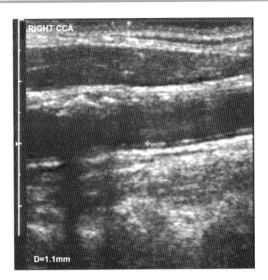

RIGHT CCA

D=1.1mm

1b Echo-bright plaque

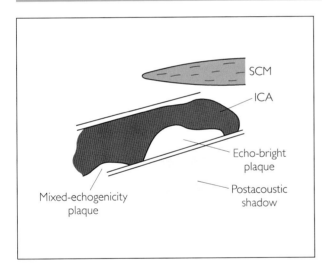

SCM

ICA

Echo-bright plaque

Postacoustic shadow

Mixed-echogenicity plaque

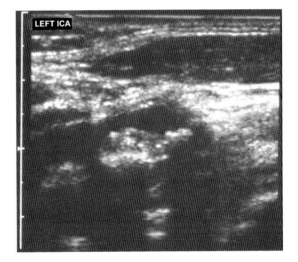

LEFT ICA

1c Echo-poor plaque

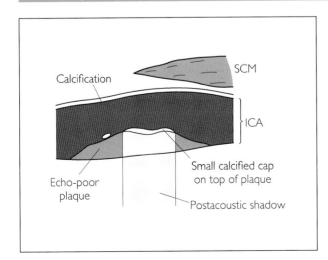

Calcification

SCM

ICA

Echo-poor plaque

Small calcified cap on top of plaque

Postacoustic shadow

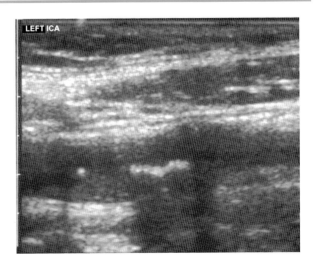

LEFT ICA

WHAT TO LOOK FOR **SCAN IMAGE**

1d Spectral Doppler 0%–49% ICA stenosis

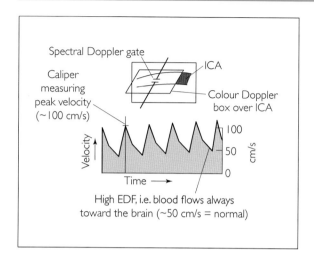

Spectral Doppler gate

Caliper measuring peak velocity (~100 cm/s)

ICA

Colour Doppler box over ICA

Velocity → | Time →

100
50
0

cm/s

High EDF, i.e. blood flows always toward the brain (~50 cm/s = normal)

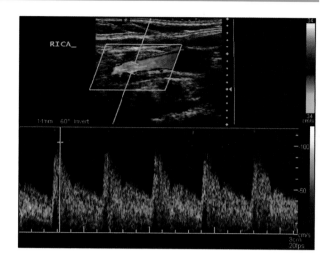

1e Spectral Doppler 50%–69% ICA stenosis

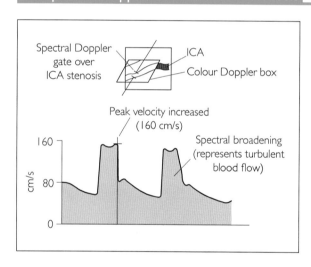

Spectral Doppler gate over ICA stenosis

ICA

Colour Doppler box

Peak velocity increased (160 cm/s)

Spectral broadening (represents turbulent blood flow)

160
80
0

cm/s

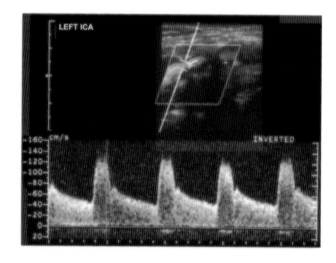

1f Spectral Doppler >70% ICA stenosis

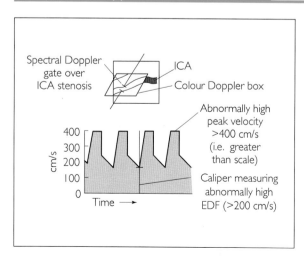

Spectral Doppler gate over ICA stenosis

ICA

Colour Doppler box

Abnormally high peak velocity >400 cm/s (i.e. greater than scale)

Caliper measuring abnormally high EDF (>200 cm/s)

400
300
200
100
0

cm/s

Time →

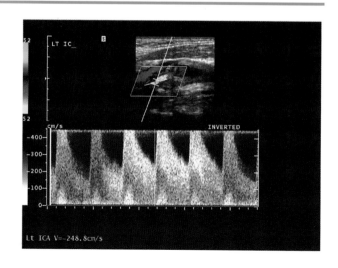

● 2 *Subclavian steal syndrome*

This is due to occlusion of the proximal subclavian (or brachiocephalic) artery— i.e. it is usually due to an occlusive atheromatous plaque. Blood flows in a *retrograde* direction down the same-side vertebral artery to supply the distal subclavian artery.

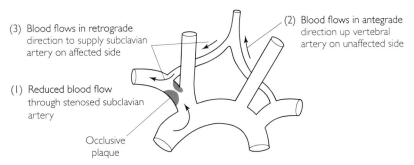

(3) Blood flows in retrograde direction to supply subclavian artery on affected side

(2) Blood flows in antegrade direction up vertebral artery on unaffected side

(1) Reduced blood flow through stenosed subclavian artery

Occlusive plaque

Ultrasound features

● Plaque seen in subclavian (or brachiocephalic) artery
● Absence of flow in subclavian (or brachiocephalic) artery with colour Doppler
● Retrograde flow in unilateral vertebral artery

WHAT TO LOOK FOR

SCAN IMAGE

2a Normal vertebral spectral Doppler

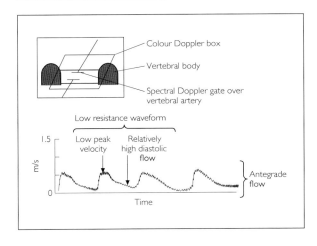

Colour Doppler box

Vertebral body

Spectral Doppler gate over vertebral artery

Low resistance waveform

Low peak velocity

Relatively high diastolic flow

Antegrade flow

Time

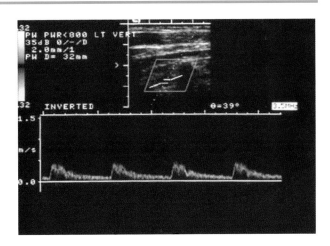

2b Partial subclavian steal spectral Doppler

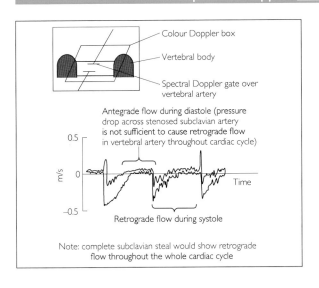

Colour Doppler box

Vertebral body

Spectral Doppler gate over vertebral artery

Antegrade flow during diastole (pressure drop across stenosed subclavian artery is not sufficient to cause retrograde flow in vertebral artery throughout cardiac cycle)

Time

Retrograde flow during systole

Note: complete subclavian steal would show retrograde flow throughout the whole cardiac cycle

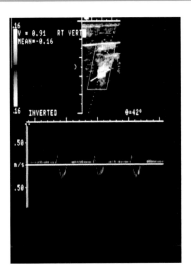

ANATOMY

(i) LS: anatomy

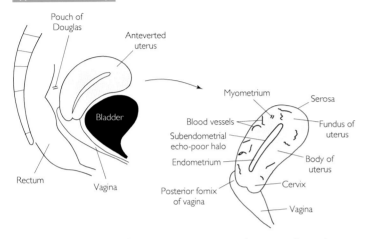

- 80% of women will have an anteverted or anteflexed uterus.
- Normal myometrium has homogenous echotexture. Fine echo-poor vessels can be seen within it.
- Endometrium is echo-bright (appearances vary with menstrual cycle – see (iv)) and surrounded by an echo-poor subendometrial halo, which represents a rim of compacted myometrium.
- It is normal to see a trace of free fluid in the Pouch of Douglas postovulation.
- Note that LS and TS ultrasound planes in the pelvis are defined in relation to the uterus, which often lies deviated to one side.
- The size of the uterus varies depending on the age of the woman and the number of pregnancies.

(ii) TS: anatomy

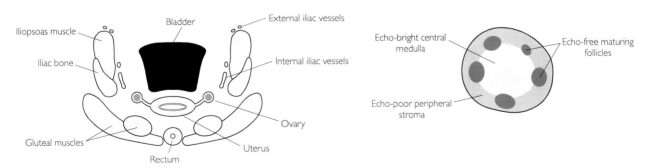

(iii) Ovary

The ovaries are attached to the uterus via the ovarian ligaments and a mobile mesovarium. As a result, they can be difficult to locate.

DOI: 10.1201/9781003381655-10

(iv) Uterine and ovarian cyclical change

	Uterine	Ovarian
Days 1–4: menstruation	Blood in cavity may cause separation of echo-bright endometrial lines	Small follicles (<5 mm)
Days 5–12: proliferation	Thin line of echo-bright endometrium thickens slowly	Dominant follicle enlarges (several follicles enlarge but one becomes dominant)
Days 13–16: peri-ovulatory	Endometrium appears echo-poor with echo-bright rim and central stripe: 'triple-line sign'	Dominant follicle ruptures
Days 17–28: secretory	Thick irregular echo-bright line	Corpus luteum appears and slowly regresses

(v) Normal uterine measurements

Uterine sizes	Length (cm)	Width (cm)	Depth (cm)	Ratio cervix: fundus (cm)
Prepubertal	3.0	1.5	1.0	2:1
Nulliparous	7.1	4.6	3.3	1:2
Multiparous	8.9	5.8	4.3	1:3
Postmenopausal	7.9	4.9	3.2	1:1

PERFORMING THE TRANSABDOMINAL SCAN

- **Patient position:** Supine.
- **Preparation:** Full bladder.
- Document LMP and take a brief gynaecological history.
- **Probe:** Low-frequency (3–5 MHz) curvilinear.
- **Machine:** Select gynaecological preset mode. Use two focal zones for imaging ovaries. Use tissue harmonics and compound imaging to improve image quality.
- **Method:** Acquire more images for each step if pathology is found.

PROBE POSITION

INSTRUCTIONS

1 LS: uterus/endometrium

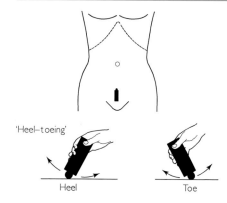

'Heel–toeing'

Heel   Toe

- Begin by placing the probe midline in the suprapubic area.
- Look for the bladder in LS with the uterus posterior to it. Tilt the probe (see below) and adjust the FOV to optimize the image. (*Hint*: Resting the end of the probe on the symphysis pubis gives good views.)
- Now look for the endometrial stripe, which varies in appearance with both age and stage of the menstrual cycle:
  - Is there any thickening or echotexture abnormalities?
  - Measure its thickness
- Acquire a representative image.

Endometrial imaging

- Try to get the transducer parallel to the uterus for optimal imaging – by 'heel–toeing' the probe – e.g. if the uterus is anteverted/anteflexed then 'heel' the probe
- Always measure thickness in LS
- Do not include any cavity fluid in the measurement
- Normal values: <15 mm premenopausal; <5 mm postmenopausal

2 LS: lateral uterus

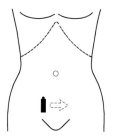

- Keep the probe in the LS position.
- Scan out towards both adnexae by tilting the probe laterally and using the bladder as a window. While doing this, observe for any fibroids or echotexture abnormalities within the myometrium.
- Acquire representative images of left and right lateral aspects of the uterus.

WHAT TO LOOK FOR

SCAN IMAGE

1

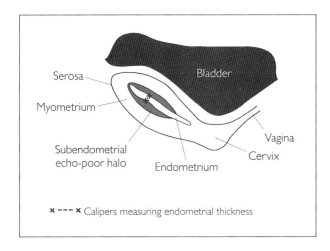

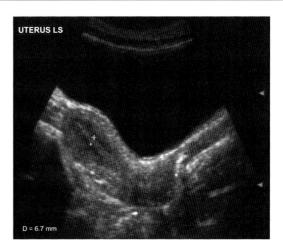

2

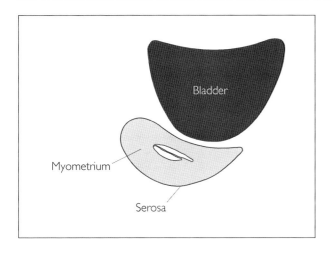

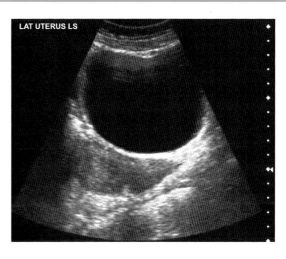

PROBE POSITION

INSTRUCTIONS

3 LS: left and right adnexae

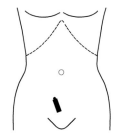

- Scan out further laterally on both sides into each adnexal region.
- Look for each ovary in LS. Narrow the FOV, and use two focal zones. The internal iliac vessels are the lateral boundaries of the pelvis and useful landmarks to help locate the ovaries.
- If bowel gas is obscuring the image, try to displace it by pressing with your free hand.
- Are there any solid or cystic adnexal lesions?
- Acquire representative images of left and right adnexae, and the ovaries if identified.

Imaging the ovary

- Optimize image: narrow FOV, increase frequency, two focal zones, use zoom
- Is it an ovary?
  - Can echo-free follicles be seen?
  - Could it be bowel? (not round in both planes and displays peristalsis)
- After menopause, the ovaries atrophy and can be hard to see. In these cases, the aim of the study is simply to exclude any adnexal masses

WHAT TO LOOK FOR

SCAN IMAGE

3a

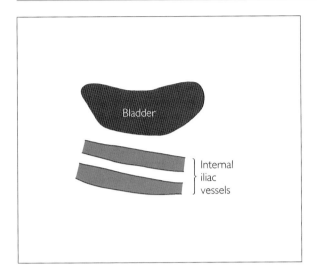

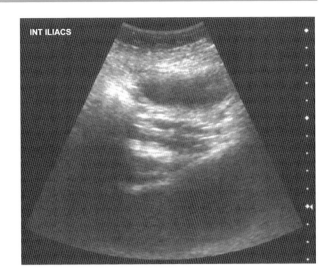

3b

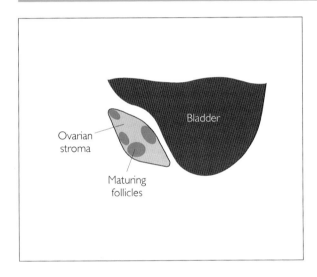

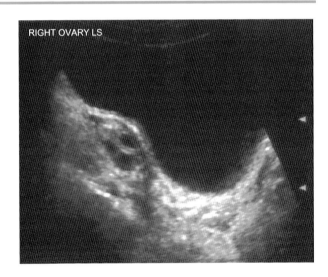

PROBE POSITION	**INSTRUCTIONS**

4 TS: uterus

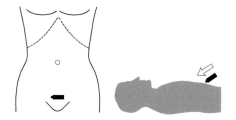

- Now turn the probe 90° anticlockwise. Look for the TS image of the bladder with the uterus/vagina posterior to it.
- Adjust the FOV and focus position.
- Scan through the uterus from vagina to fundus by tilting the probe superiorly and inferiorly.
- Acquire representative images (e.g. of fundus/body/cervix).

5 TS: left and right adnexae

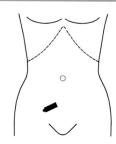

- Scan out into each adnexa by tilting the probe laterally and using the bladder as a window.
- Look for each ovary in TS. Narrow the FOV, and use two focal zones. The widest portion of the uterine body is a useful landmark to help locate the ovaries.
- Acquire representative images of left and right adnexae, and the ovaries if identified.

Complete the scan by imaging both kidneys as per Chapter 4 (looking for hydronephrosis from malignant ureteric obstruction)

WHAT TO LOOK FOR

SCAN IMAGE

4

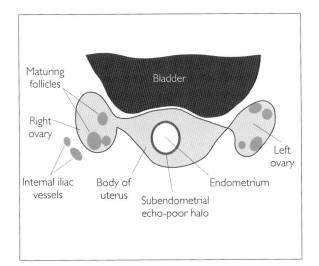

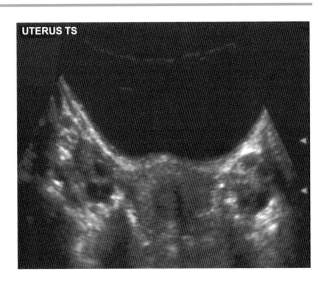

UTERUS TS

5

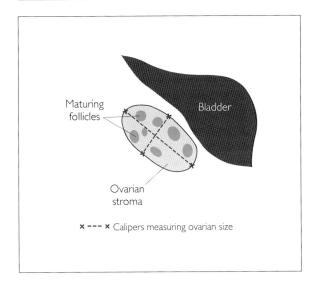

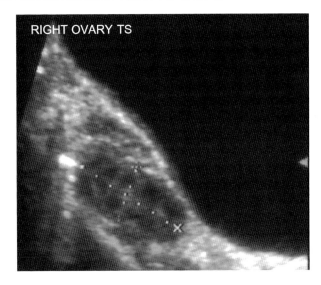

RIGHT OVARY TS

TRANSVAGINAL (TV) ANATOMY

(i) LS

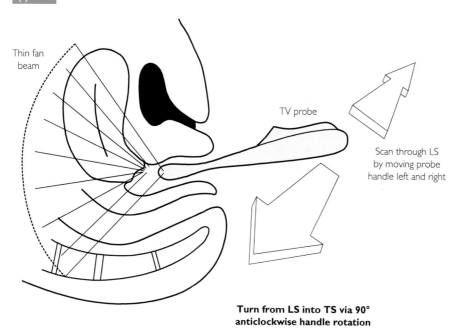

Thin fan beam

TV probe

Scan through LS by moving probe handle left and right

Turn from LS into TS via 90° anticlockwise handle rotation

(ii) TS

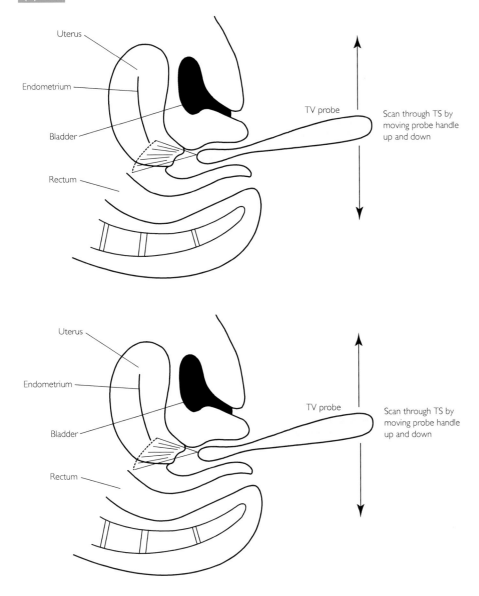

These are the two basic imaging planes employed in TV scanning. Remember that the fan beam is thin and that to scan through structures, the operator needs to move the probe in LS, TS and oblique planes.

PERFORMING THE TRANSVAGINAL SCAN

- It is advised that a chaperone be present during the examination. Explain the nature of the examination, asking for consent.
- **Patient position:** Supine with legs abducted, knees flexed, and pad under buttocks or with buttocks at end of couch and feet supported on a chair.
- **Preparation:** Empty bladder.
- Document LMP and take a brief gynaecological history. Always ask if any area in the pelvis is particularly tender.
- **Probe:** Select TV probe and apply probe cover with gel.
- **Machine:** Select TV gynaecological preset mode. Use two focal zones for imaging the ovaries. Use compound imaging to improve image quality.
- **Method:** Acquire more than just the representative images for each step if pathology is found.

PROBE POSITION	INSTRUCTIONS

1 LS: uterus/endometrium

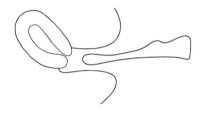

- Begin by inserting the TV probe until resistance is felt.
- Look for the uterus LS. The probe/cervix interface will be at the top of the screen, with the fan beam coming down. An anteverted uterus appears on the left side of the screen and a retroverted uterus on the right.
- Now look for the endometrial stripe, which varies in appearance with both age and stage of the menstrual cycle:
  - Is there any thickening or echotexture abnormality?
  - Measure its thickness.
- Acquire a representative image.

2 LS: lateral uterus

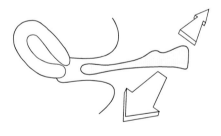

- Keep the probe in the LS position.
- Scan out through the body of the uterus towards both adnexae in the LS plane, by tilting the probe handle to the left and right. While doing this, observe for any fibroids or echotexture abnormalities within the myometrium.
- Acquire representative images of left and right lateral aspects of the uterus.

3 LS: left and right adnexae

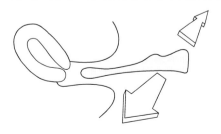

- Tilt the probe handle more laterally now into each adnexal region.
- Look for each ovary in LS. Narrow the FOV, and use two focal zones. The internal iliac vessels are the lateral boundaries of the pelvis, and are useful landmarks to help locate the ovaries.
- If bowel gas shadows interfere try displacing it by pressing with your free hand.
- Are there any solid or cystic adnexal lesions?
- Acquire representative images of left and right adnexae, and the ovaries if identified.

WHAT TO LOOK FOR

SCAN IMAGE

1

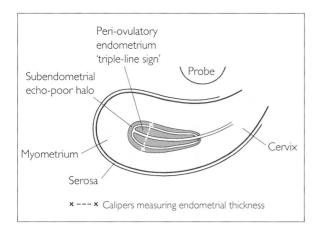

Peri-ovulatory
endometrium
'triple-line sign'

Probe

Subendometrial
echo-poor halo

Myometrium

Cervix

Serosa

x - - - x Calipers measuring endometrial thickness

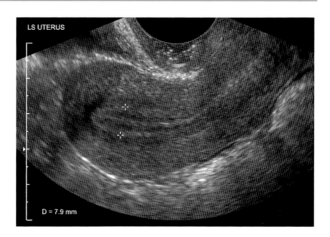

LS UTERUS

D = 7.9 mm

2

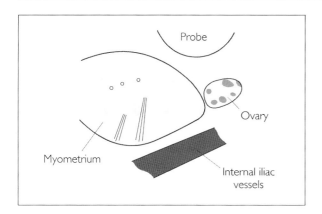

Probe

Ovary

Myometrium

Internal iliac
vessels

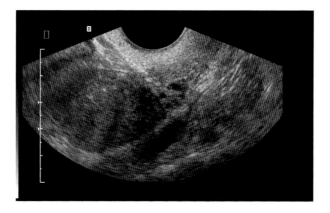

3

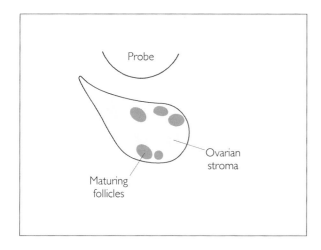

Probe

Ovarian
stroma

Maturing
follicles

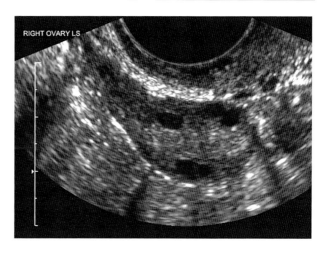

RIGHT OVARY LS

PROBE POSITION	**INSTRUCTIONS**

4 TS: uterus

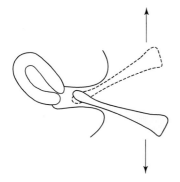

- Now turn the probe handle 90° anticlockwise (withdraw it slightly first to avoid catching the cervix).
- Look for a TS image of the uterus.
- Adjust the FOV and focus position.
- Scan through the uterus from cervix to fundus. For an anteverted uterus, tilting the probe handle down (tip pointing up) will show the fundus. Tilt the tip down to look for the cervix. *Hint:* If the bed restricts the full range of probe movement, ask the patient to tilt the pelvis up.
- Acquire representative images (e.g., of fundus/body/cervix).

5 TS: left and right adnexae

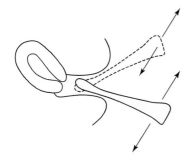

- Scan out into each adnexa by tilting the probe handle contralaterally.
- Look for each ovary in TS. Narrow the FOV, and use two focal zones. The widest portion of the uterine body is a useful landmark to help locate the ovaries.
- Acquire representative images of left and right adnexae, and the ovaries if identified.

Visceral slide assessment

The pelvic organs should normally move freely over each other on deep respiration and manual palpation (i.e. between hand and probe). If this does not occur, it may indicate inflammatory or malignant pathology.

● *Polycystic ovarian syndrome protocol*

- The role of ultrasound is to look for evidence of polycystic ovaries. Polycystic ovarian syndrome (PCOS) diagnosis requires the assimilation of clinical, biochemical and ultrasound findings.
- It is necessary to measure the ovarian volumes (a TV scan gives more accuracy than a TA scan).
- Calculate from LS and TS images, measuring the diameter in three planes. The split screen function can be helpful for this.
- Use the measurement package to calculate the volume (on most machines).
- Normal volume $<10\,cm^3$ in premenopausal women.
- See the pathology section for more on this.

WHAT TO LOOK FOR

SCAN IMAGE

4

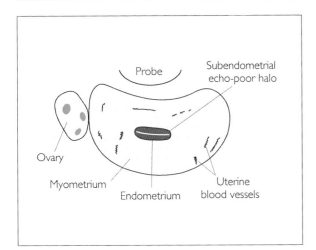

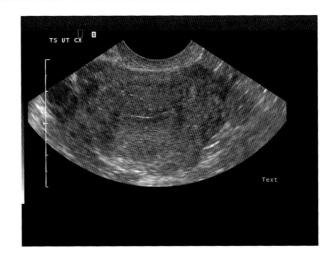

5

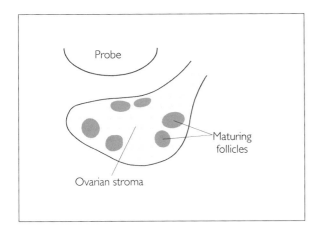

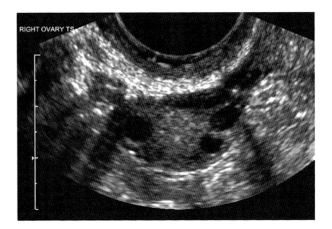

Measurement of ovary

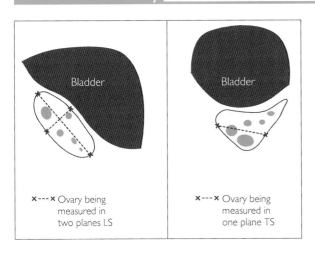

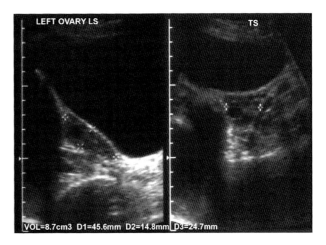

PATHOLOGY

● 1 *Uterine fibroids (leiomyoma)*

These are a very common finding (25% of premenopausal women). Fibroids are benign smooth muscle tumours with a fibrous element. They are oestrogen-dependent: can grow rapidly during pregnancy, and tend to regress after the menopause. They are often asymptomatic, but can cause menorrhagia, pain or subfertility, depending on their size and location:

- mural: arise within the myometrium (95% of fibroids)
- submucosal: protrude into the endometrial cavity
- subserosal: project from the uterine surface

Ultrasound features
- Focal uterine enlargement
- Well-defined echo-poor mass with characteristic lamellated/whirled internal echo pattern
- May contain echo-bright areas of calcification or degeneration.

Diffuse enlargement of the uterus without a focal mass is more likely to be adenomyosis – look for small cystic spaces in the myometrium and asymmetry of the anterior and posterior wall thickness.

● 2 Nabothian cysts

These are small benign inclusion cysts, which can be seen in the region of the endocervical canal. Clinically, they are most commonly seen on the surface of the cervix. They are of no clinical significance.

Ultrasound features
- Smooth edge
- Thin wall
- Echo-free contents
- Postacoustic enhancement

● 3 Polycystic ovarian syndrome

PCOS is diagnosed based on clinical, biochemical and ultrasound findings. Only about 50% of PCOS patients will have the typical ultrasound findings. The absence of these therefore does not preclude the diagnosis. Conversely, approximately 25% of Caucasian women and 33% of Indian women will have a polycystic ovary but without the syndrome.

Ultrasound features (Rotterdam criteria)
- Ovarian volume is usually >10 cm3
- 2 immature follicles (3–9 mm) in the ovary. Other authorities advise using >25 follicles
- Peripheral ovarian stroma is echo-bright and of increased volume

Hint: PCOS is not to be confused with multicystic ovaries, which are seen at the menarche and in anorexia (normal ovarian volumes, less numerous larger follicles).

WHAT TO LOOK FOR

SCAN IMAGE

1 Uterine fibroid

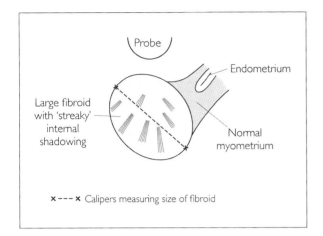

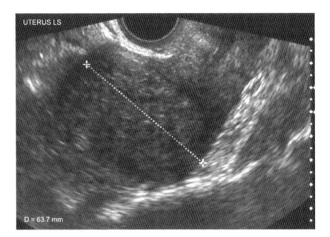

Hint: Note the 'claw sign' where the myometrium has a claw-like shape as it stretches around the fibroid. Confirms it is uterine in origin.

2 Nabothian cysts

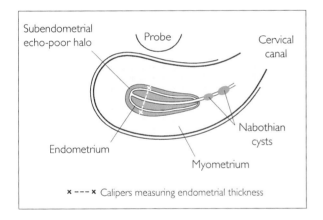

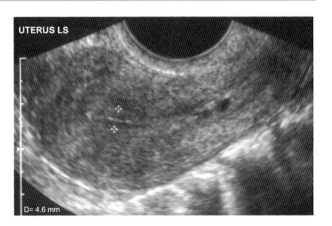

3 PCOS

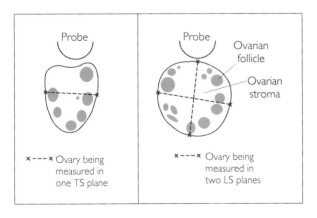

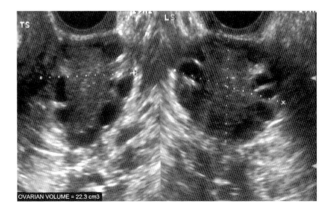

● 4 Ovarian cysts

When an ovarian lesion is identified, it is important to classify its appearance as benign, suspicious or malignant. This will determine if follow-up is required.

(a) Benign

These display the typical features of a simple cyst (see previous pages)

They measure <3 cm in a premenopausal woman; <5 cm in a postmenopausal woman. They are usually physiological (e.g. follicular cysts). They are very common and of no clinical significance. They do not need to be followed up. If a lesion is recognized by the operator as a dominant follicle or a corpus luteum, it is advised to report them as such and avoid the word, 'cyst', which may cause unnecessary alarm.

(b) Suspicious

These are cysts that have a more complex appearance, often caused by internal haemorrhage. Suspicious features include:

- large size: >3 cm in a premenopausal woman; >5 cm in a postmenopausal woman
- internal echoes
- fine internal septations
- Consider using the 'IOTA simple rules' if unsure. https://iota.education

A follow-up scan is needed in 6–8 weeks (to check for size reduction/resolution).

(c) Malignant

These cystic lesions have a frankly neoplastic appearance. They are usually due to primary *ovarian cancer. Features suggestive of malignancy include:*

- thick irregular walls
- thick internal septations
- internal echoes
- papillary nodules on cyst wall
- usually >5 cm

Look for other malignant features:

- hydronephrosis
- liver metastases
- omental cake
- ascites
- pleural effusions
- peritoneal deposits

WHAT TO LOOK FOR   **SCAN IMAGE**

4a Simple ovarian cyst

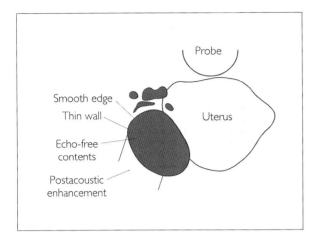

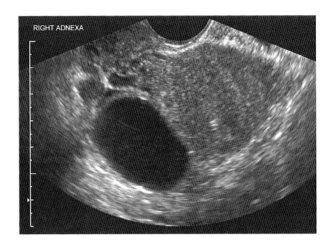

4b Complex ovarian cyst

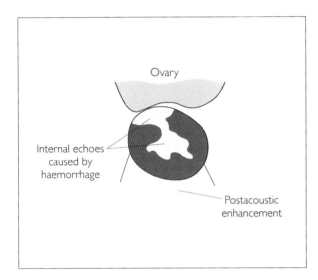

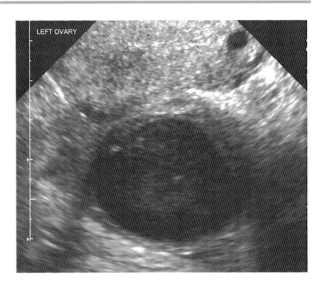

4c Ovarian malignancy

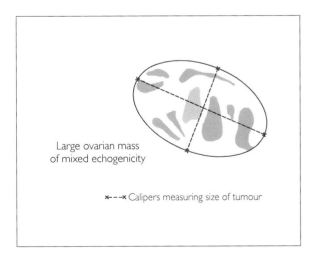

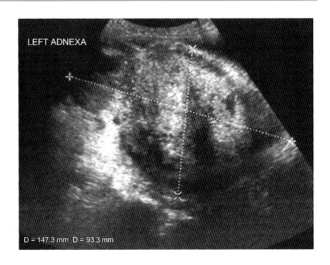

● 5 *Endometrial thickening*

The endometrium is considered thickened on ultrasound if:

- > 5 mm in a premenopausal woman
- > mm in a postmenopausal woman

(a) Focal thickening

This can be caused by an endometrial polyp or submucosal fibroid.

Conspicuity of a polyp will change during a menstrual cycle. It will be most clear against the lower echo proliferative endometrium and harder to see or hidden within the higher echo secretory endometrium.

(b) Diffuse thickening

- Endometrial hyperplasia:
  - physiological
  - drug-induced (tamoxifen, HRT)
  - oestrogen-secreting tumours
- Endometrial carcinoma:
  - this can arise from hyperplasia or occur de novo
  - it is a common malignancy in postmenopausal women. Ultrasound cannot reliably distinguish between hyperplasia and carcinoma, so hysteroscopy and biopsy are required in all cases.

(c) Features suspicious of malignancy

- Thickened endometrium with irregular margin
- Endometrial mass of mixed echogenicity
- Endometrial mass seen to be infiltrating into the myometrium
- Extrauterine deposits

WHAT TO LOOK FOR

SCAN IMAGE

5a Focal thickening

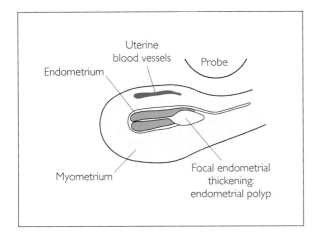

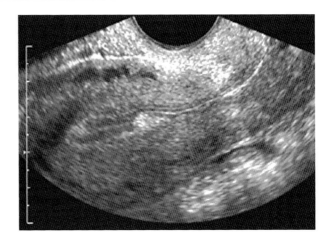

5b Diffuse thickening

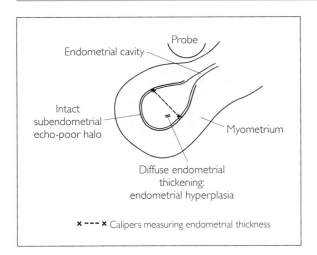

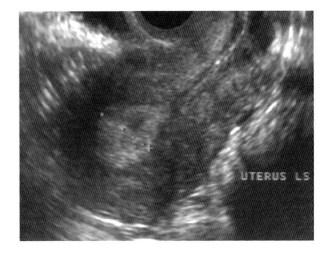

5c Malignant thickening

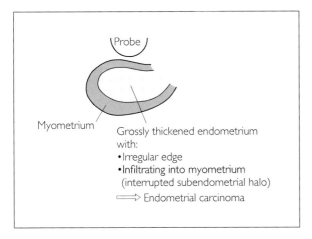

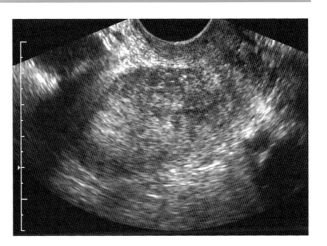

● 6 *Intrauterine device*

Some coils can be harder to see than others, and it may only be possible to see their endpoints. To be effective, they must be positioned <5 mm from the upper end of the endometrial cavity.

Ultrasound features
- Usually identified as a hyperechoic structure within the cavity
- Casts a strong acoustic shadow
- The acoustic shadow is most pronounced when imaged in TS as the coil crosses the full width of the ultrasound beam. When imaged in LS the coil may only take up a small part of the beam width meaning its shadow is less.
- Check the intrauterine device (IUD) is not embedded in the myometrium.

● 7 *False pelvic mass*

A mirror-image artefact of the bladder is seen posterior to the uterus. It can easily be mistaken for a pelvic mass. It is caused by the reflection of the beam from bowel loops in the pouch of Douglas.

Ultrasound features
- Lack of well-defined superior and inferior walls of the 'mass'
- The 'mass' is located too far posteriorly to be anatomically possible

In slim patients, beware the sacrum!

WHAT TO LOOK FOR   **SCAN IMAGE**

6 IUD

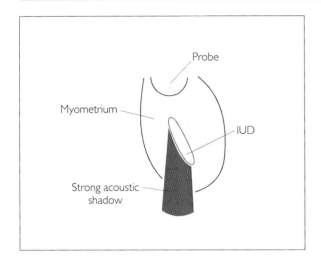

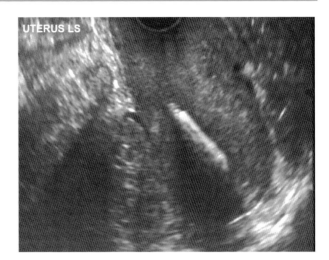

7 False pelvic mass

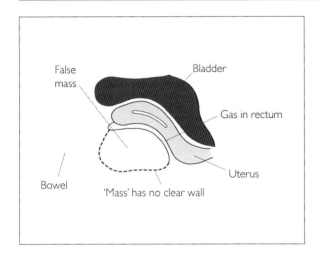

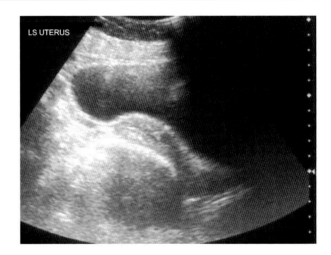

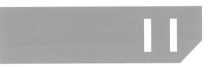

Early pregnancy

USEFUL ANATOMY

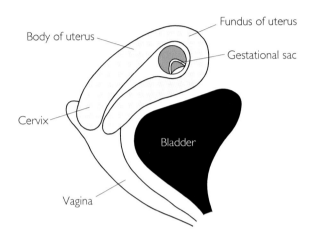

5¹/₂ weeks' gestation

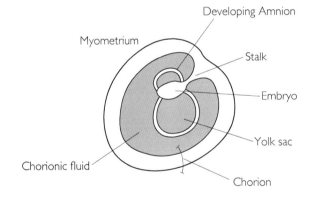

Later

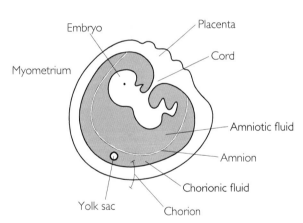

● *Key points*

- 80% of women have an anteverted or anteflexed uterus.
- The gestational sac is usually sited in the fundal region of the uterus.
- The yolk sac is normally the first structure to be seen within the gestational sac. Its presence confirms that this is a gestation and not just a fluid collection.

DOI: 10.1201/9781003381655-11

PERFORMING THE SCAN

The primary role of ultrasound in the first trimester of pregnancy is to confirm the presence of a live intrauterine pregnancy and to distinguish this from a pregnancy that will not progress or ectopic pregnancy.

Appropriate medical and nursing support must be available, and there should be access to a quiet side room when bad news is given. Allow partners to be present during the scan. It is advised that a chaperone should always be present (essential for male examiners). Begin by explaining the nature of the examination and the reasons for doing it, asking the patient for verbal consent. Take a brief obstetric history, and document dates of the LMP and pregnancy test.

The scan can be performed either transabdominally or transvaginally.

● Transabdominal scan

- **Patient position:** Supine.
- **Preparation:** In thin patients, a full bladder is not always needed. Provided that the uterus is anteverted, good visualization of its contents can usually be achieved.
- **Probe:** Low-frequency (3–5 MHz) curvilinear.
- **Machine:** Select early pregnancy or obstetric preset mode, and use two focal zones. Use tissue harmonics and compound imaging to improve image quality.

● Transvaginal scan

- **Patient position:** Supine with legs abducted (see Chapter 10).
- **Preparation:** Empty bladder.
- **Probe:** Select TV probe and apply probe cover with gel.
- **Machine:** Select early pregnancy or gynaecological preset mode, compound imaging and use two focal zones.

The scanning techniques are basically the same as those used in a regular gynaecological scan. Reference should be made to Chapter 10.

● Safe practice

- The mechanical index (MI) and thermal index (TI) should be kept to the lowest level that still allows an image to be achieved: it is recommended that an MI < 0.7 be used.
- Minimize exposure of the foetus by using the freeze and ciné loop functions to reduce the scan time.
- Use the as low as reasonably acceptable (ALARA) principle when doing early pregnancy scans.
- Colour and/or spectral Doppler of the foetus should usually be avoided in the first trimester.

Early-pregnancy reporting

The report should normally include the following information:

- Gestational sac position: is it intrauterine?
- Foetal number.
- If the pregnancy is multifetal, indicate the number of placentae (chorionicity).
- Foetal heart pulsation: present/absent?
- Mean sac diameter (MSD) or if present, CRL/HC.
- Estimated gestational age and which measurement was used for this.
- If no embryo is seen, the presence or absence of the yolk sac should be indicated.
- Include a description of any gynaecological masses that are present.

Several terms are used to conclude the report of a pregnancy that is not ongoing. These include missed miscarriage and failed pregnancy ('failed' is a word that many patients dislike). Many also use 'missed miss' to cover everything, including anembryonic pregnancy. It is recommended that each department agree on a common terminology.

PROBE POSITION

INSTRUCTIONS

1 LS: uterus/gestational sac

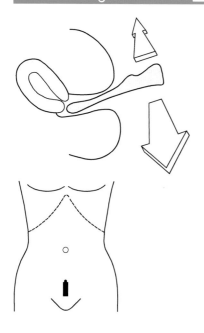

- For either TA or TV method, begin by imaging the uterus in the LS plane. Initially use the widest FOV. Adjust the depth and focus position (for more details, see Chapter 10).
- Look for an intrauterine gestational sac, and if present, observe:
  - if it contains a visible yolk sac or embryo(s)
  - if any heart pulsations can be seen
  - the relationship of the sac to the cervix
- It may help to narrow the FOV and use zoom
- Acquire a representative image.
- Notice how the TV scan in 1b gives much greater clarity about the gestation sac contents than the TA scan in 1a.

Foetal heart pulsation

- This should definitely be visible when the crown–rump length (CRL) is measured as >7mm via a TV scan or >10mm via TA.
- Heart pulsations may be detected with CRLs as low as 3mm.

Time-motion (M-mode)

- M-mode imparts less ultrasound energy into the embryo than colour or spectral Doppler
- Now formally assess for a foetal heart pulsation in real time:
  - select M-mode function
  - on most machines, a dual image will appear (a real-time image and an M-mode image)
  - place the M-mode line across the estimated position of the foetal chest
  - look for M-mode evidence of heart pulsation
- Acquire a representative image.

Foetus

- Now measure:
  - gestational sac size
  - CRL and/or
  - head circumference (see below for more details)
- Acquire representative images.

WHAT TO LOOK FOR   **SCAN IMAGE**

1a LS: uterus TA

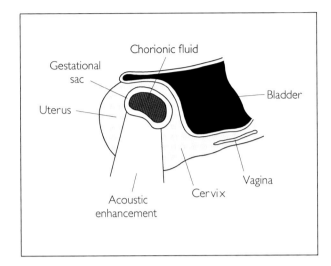

Chorionic fluid
Gestational sac
Uterus
Bladder
Acoustic enhancement
Cervix
Vagina

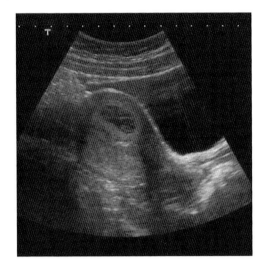

1b LS: uterus TV

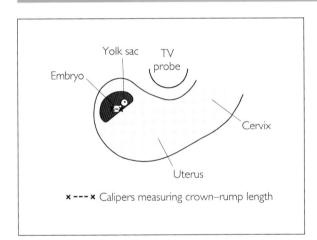

Yolk sac
TV probe
Embryo
Cervix
Uterus

×---× Calipers measuring crown–rump length

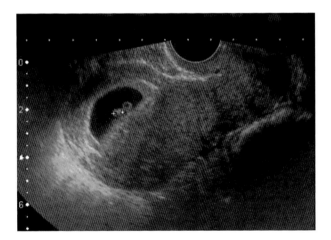

1c TS: time–motion mode

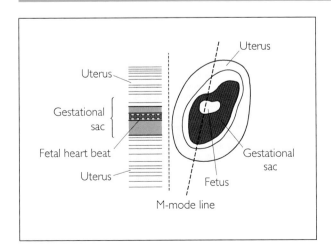

Uterus
Uterus
Gestational sac
Fetal heart beat
Uterus
Gestational sac
Fetus
M-mode line

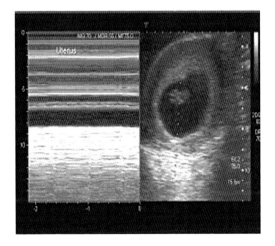

PROBE POSITION	**INSTRUCTIONS**

2 TS: uterus/gestational sac

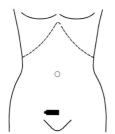

- Now image the uterus in the TS plane via a 90° anticlockwise probe rotation for both TV and TA methods (for more details, see Chapter 10).
- Scan through the uterus from the cervix to fundus:
  - again looking for an intrauterine gestational sac
  - when doing this, remember to check for any fibroids or echotexture abnormalities within the myometrium
- Acquire a representative image.

3 LS/TS: left and right adnexae

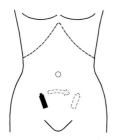

- When performing a pregnancy scan, it is good practice to also examine the ovaries and adnexal regions for pathology.
- Scan out towards both adnexae in the LS and TS planes by angling the probe laterally for both TV and TA methods (for more details, see Chapter 10).
- In particular, look for any signs to suggest an ectopic pregnancy (see pathology section).
- Acquire representative images of left and right adnexae, and the ovaries if identified.

ESTIMATING GESTATIONAL AGE

There are several ways in which this can be done, and three commonly used methods are discussed below. Note that using a TV scanning method will permit more accurate estimations.

● 1 Gestational sac size

- If a gestational sac is detected, the mean sac diameter (MSD) can be used to estimate the gestational age of the embryo.
- Calculate the MSD using one LS and one TS image and measure the sac diameter in three orthogonal planes. The split screen function can be helpful for this.
- Add all three measurements together and divide by 3: this is the MSD (in millimetres).
- Acquire a representative image.
- By cross-reference with special charts, the MSD can be used to estimate the gestational age of the embryo.

WHAT TO LOOK FOR   **SCAN IMAGE**

2 TS: uterus

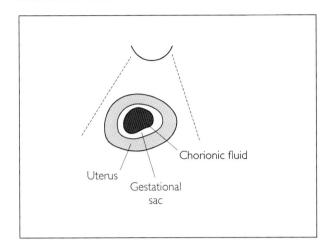

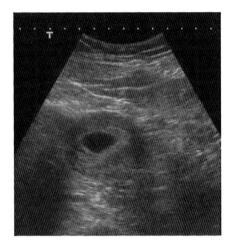

3 TS: adnexae

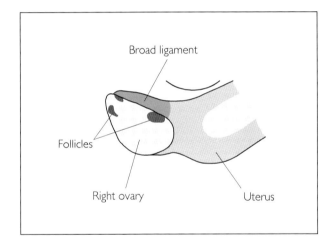

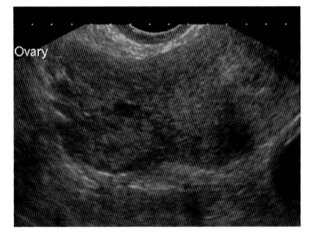

1 Measurement: gestational sac

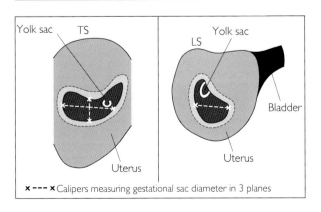

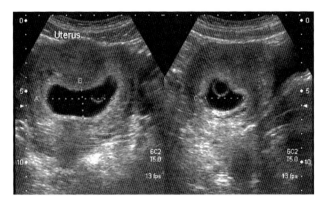

● *2 Crown–rump length*

- If an embryo is detected within the gestational sac, its CRL should be used to estimate gestational age.
- First optimize the image for accuracy of measurement: narrow the FOV, use multiple focal zones and use the zoom function.
- The embryo should be measured in its longest axis, which is found by gentle probe rotation in LS, TS and oblique planes.
- When found, freeze the image.
- Select the CRL measurement package (on most machines).
- Place one calliper at the upper end of the embryo (its crown) and another at the lower end (its rump).
- The machine will display an estimated gestational age (if this function is not available, the distance can be cross-referenced with a special CRL chart).

Hint: Primitive rhomboencephalon can make the head look like a yolk sac. Common mistakes include omitting the head or including the yolk sac in the measurement!

● *3 Head circumference (HC)*

- If an embryo's gestational age has been estimated at 13 weeks or more by CRL then HC should be used to give a more accurate estimation.
- First optimize the image: narrow the FOV, use multiple focal zones and use the zoom function.
- For standardized, reproducible results, the head should be measured in a true axial (TS) plane.
- Find this via fine manipulation of the probe, looking for the following key anatomical landmarks:
    - ugby ball'-shaped head
    - interhemispheric fissure (IHF)
    - equal hemisphere diameters
    - thalamus
    - cavum septum pellucidum
    - anterior horns of the lateral ventricles
- Select the HC measurement package (on most machines).
- Measure the outer skull bone surface.
- The machine will display an estimated gestational age (if this function is not available, the distance can be cross-referenced with a special HC chart).

WHAT TO LOOK FOR　　　　　　　**SCAN IMAGE**

2a Measurement: CRL

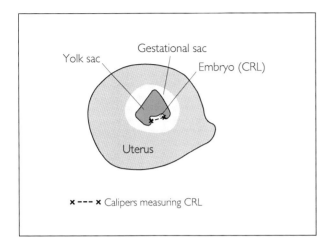

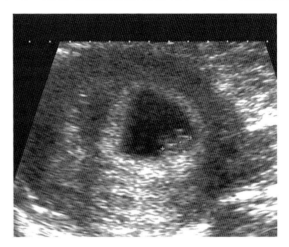

2b Measurement: CRL

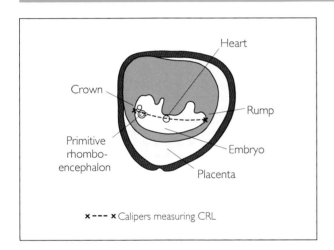

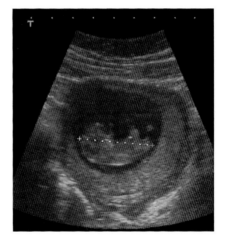

3 Measurement: foetal head

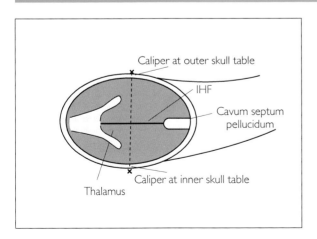

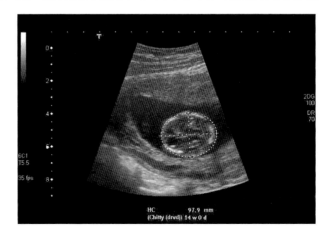

EARLY PREGNANCY ANOMALIES

● 1 Multifetal pregnancy

- State the presence/absence and thickness of the septum.
- Assess the number of placentae (chorionicity): look for the lambda sign (placental tissue forming in the septum between the embryos). The lambda sign indicates a dichorionic diamniotic pregnancy.
- Assess the number of amniotic cavities (amnionicity).
- Indicate on the report whether the pregnancy is monochorionic/monoamniotic, monochorionic/diamniotic or dichorionic/diamniotic.
- Note the relative position of the foetuses.
- If possible, assess whether the foetuses are of the same sex.
- A diagram of the foetuses on the report is helpful and will assist in subsequent scans.

● 2 Corpus luteal cyst of pregnancy

Following fertilization, the corpus luteum persists (due to β-HCG). In this condition bleeding occurs into it, often causing pain. Most resolve spontaneously.

Ultrasound features

- Most are <5 cm in size
- Thin wall
- Display internal echoes from the blood
- This complex appearance can mimic an ovarian malignancy; if there is any doubt, repeat the scan in 6–8 weeks' time (see Chapter 10 for more on ovarian cysts)

● 3 Subchorionic haemorrhage

This is venous bleeding into the subchorionic space extending to the margin of the placenta. It usually occurs in early pregnancy and is associated with smoking. It has a favourable prognosis.

Ultrasound features

- The marginal edge of the placenta is separated from the myometrium
- If the bleed is recent, it may contain internal echoes – old bleeds are echo-free

Hint: Large retroplacental haemorrhage (abruption) tends to occur in late pregnancy and has a poor outcome. It is not reliably diagnosed by ultrasound.

WHAT TO LOOK FOR   **SCAN IMAGE**

1 Dichorionic pregnancy: lambda sign

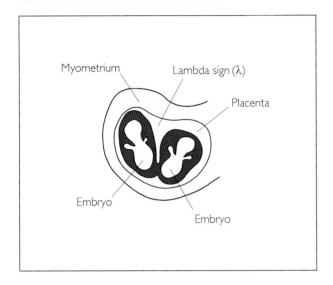

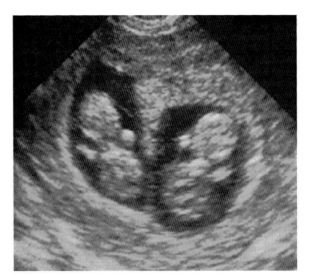

2 Corpus luteum of pregnancy

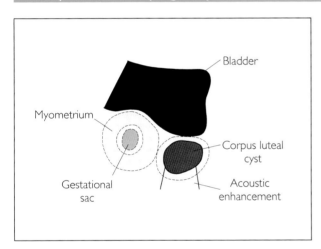

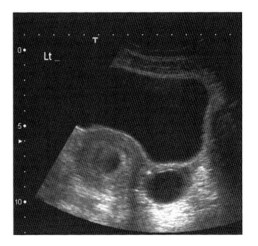

3 Subchorionic haemorrhage

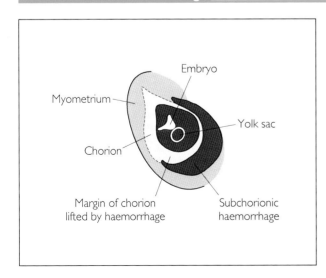

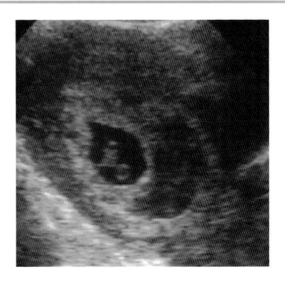

● 4 Incomplete miscarriage/retained products of conception (RPOC)

This is when fetal death occurs and some placental/fetal tissue remains within the endometrial cavity, usually causing heavy bleeding.

Do not always assume that debris in the endometrial cavity is due to RPOC. Relate the findings to any prior scans. If the patient has previously been shown to have had an intrauterine gestational sac/embryo, then the diagnosis can be made confidently. Otherwise:

- If the β-hCG level is falling, then the report should indicate that RPOC is the most likely cause
- If the β-hCG level is unknown, then an ectopic pregnancy with an associated decidual reaction is possible.

Ultrasound features
- Echo-bright or heterogeneous material is seen within the endometrial cavity

● 5 Hydatidiform mole

This rare but important condition occurs in early pregnancy and is caused by trophoblastic tissue in the placenta undergoing excessive proliferation. Occasionally, fetal tissue forms, but this is non-viable. Patients present with first-trimester bleeding and hyperemesis caused by very elevated β-hCG levels. Most hydatidiform moles are now diagnosed at pathology of the products without any prior recognizable ultrasound signs.

Treatment involves referral to a specialist centre for evacuation of uterine contents and serial monitoring of β-hCG levels to ensure complete regression. Approximately 10% will develop an invasive mole or malignant choriocarcinoma (persistently elevated β-hCG levels) and the treatment is with chemotherapy. The prognosis is generally good.

Ultrasound features
- In the early stages, the uterus is enlarged and filled with echo-bright material: 'snowstorm' appearance
- As the mole progresses, easily visible echo-poor cystic spaces develop within it: 'bunch of grapes' appearance
- Associated with large ovarian theca-lutein cysts (due to excessive β-hCG stimulation)

WHAT TO LOOK FOR **SCAN IMAGE**

4 RPOC

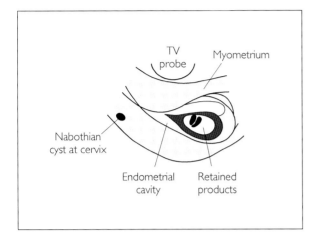

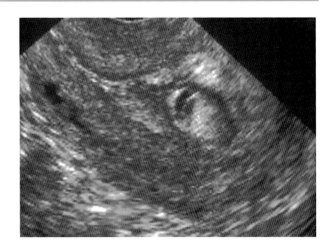

5 Hydatidiform mole

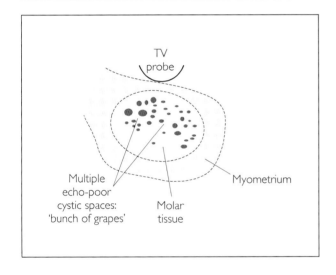

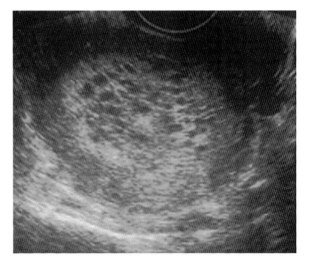

● 6 *Embryonic demise*

The following are signs of fetal death (see also NICE guideline NG126; 23.08.2023):

6a Empty sac sign
- A gestational sac, MSD >25 mm (TA or TV) with no visible yolk sac
- A gestational sac, MSD >25 mm (TA or TV) with no visible embryo

Causes of an empty sac:

- missed miscarriage
- anembryonic pregnancy
- pseudogestational sac from an ectopic pregnancy

6b Empty-amnion sign
- An amnion is clearly visible without the presence of an embryo

6c Absent fetal heart pulsation
- Embryo with a CRL >10 mm, TA with no detectable heart pulsation
- Embryo with a CRL >7 mm, TV with no detectable heart pulsation
- Flat M-mode trace

Safe diagnosis requires the independent observation of two qualified ultrasound practitioners. If either of the practitioners is in doubt, a rescan in 7–10 days is required. If a second practitioner is not available, the patient should be informed of the first practitioner's findings and offered the choice of proceeding to management or waiting for a second opinion on another day.

Note: Proceeding to management means accepting the diagnosis of miscarriage and then choosing either expectant management or evacuation. Most places prefer expectant management.

6d Failure of interval growth
- Allowing for interobserver variation, a failed pregnancy can be confirmed if there has been no growth of the MSD after a 1-week interval

WHAT TO LOOK FOR

SCAN IMAGE

6 Embryonic demise

6a Empty sac

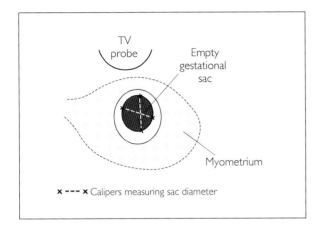

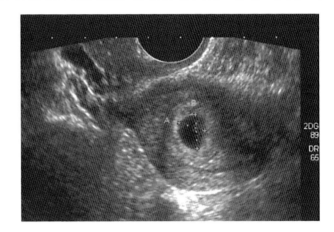

6b Empty-amnion sign

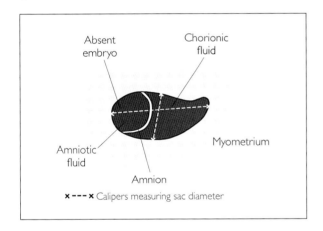

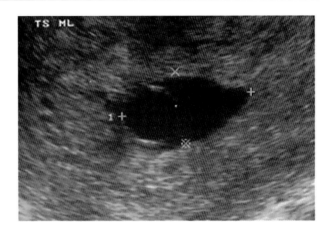

6c Absent fetal heart pulsation

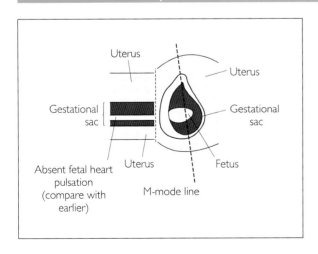

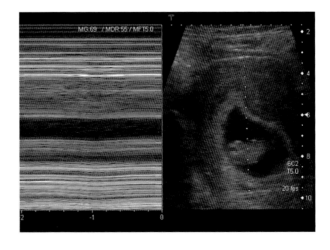

● 7 Ectopic pregnancy

This is the implantation of a pregnancy outside the endometrial cavity.

- The incidence is 0.3%–1.6% of all pregnancies and accounts for 10% of maternal deaths.
- If the patient is collapsed or there is a high clinical suspicion of ectopic pregnancy, ultrasound is not appropriate. Refer to gynaecologist urgently
- Referrals for ectopic pregnancy should have both TA and TV scans.
- The role of ultrasound is to attempt to localize the pregnancy.
- If an intrauterine pregnancy is found, an ectopic pregnancy is virtually excluded because the combination of intrauterine and ectopic pregnancy is extremely rare in normal conceptions (1 in 30000).
- In women with the following risk factors, the ectopic rate is much higher: IUD, PID, previous ectopic and tubal surgery, reversal of sterilization, infertility treatment and smoking.
- Beware a pseudogestational sac caused by decidual reaction.
- The ultrasound findings must be correlated with the clinical symptoms and β-hCG levels:
  - An empty uterus and a positive pregnancy test can be due to an intrauterine pregnancy less than 5 weeks, a miscarriage (need to have seen an intrauterine pregnancy before this examination) or an ectopic pregnancy.
  - Some centres use a discriminatory value for β-hCG >1000 mIu/ml, at which level an embryo should always be visible.

In infertility treatment, a high level of β-hCG can cause overstimulation of the ovaries and multiple large functional cysts with a large amount of pelvic fluid and pleural effusions.

Pregnancy of unknown location applies with a positive pregnancy test and no 'visible' intrauterine pregnancy and incorporates three clear possibilities: (i) Intrauterine pregnancy but too early to see; (ii) Pregnancy already miscarried but pregnancy test still positive; (iii) Ectopic pregnancy.

Ultrasound features
Pseudosac or gestation sac?
A true gestation sac:

- Lies within the endometrium and not the cavity so usually looks eccentrically placed
- Is usually more rounded
- Often has a bright rim – the chorionic rim sign
- May show the double decidual sac sign of a bright chorionic rim and a bright rim of decidua (endometrium)
- Contains embryonic structures (yolk sac or fetal pole)

A pseudo sac (false sac)

- Lies in the cavity
- Often more elongated and conforms to endometrial cavity
- No bright rim
- No embryonic structures

Ultrasound features of an ectopic pregnancy
- Free fluid in POD seen in 20%–25% of cases; hyperechoic fluid may represent blood from a ruptured ectopic
- Demonstration of an extrauterine embryonic heartbeat is diagnostic, but this is not a common finding
- The presence of free fluid containing echoes (haemoperitoneum) has a strong positive predictive value (best seen using TV method)
- Echo-bright endometrial thickening from hormonal stimulation by the ectopic is common; a pseudogestational sac is seen in 20%

A solid/cystic adnexal mass may be seen. This often has a concentric appearance to it, and has been likened to a 'doughnut'

WHAT TO LOOK FOR   **SCAN IMAGE**

7a Ectopic pregnancy: haemoperitoneum

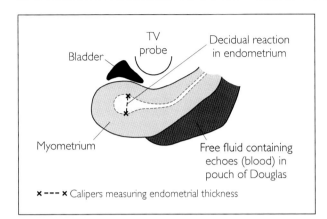

Bladder

TV probe

Decidual reaction in endometrium

Myometrium

Free fluid containing echoes (blood) in pouch of Douglas

x - - - x Calipers measuring endometrial thickness

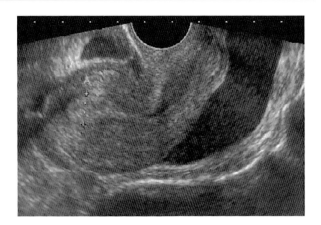

7b Ectopic pregnancy: adnexal mass

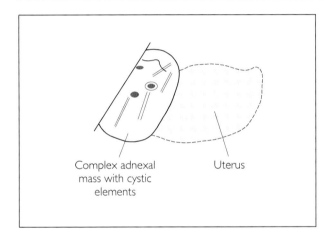

Complex adnexal mass with cystic elements

Uterus

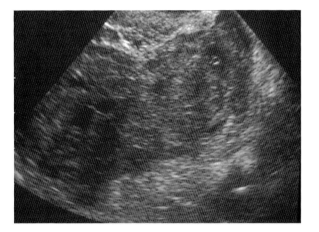

7c Ectopic pregnancy: extrauterine gestational sac

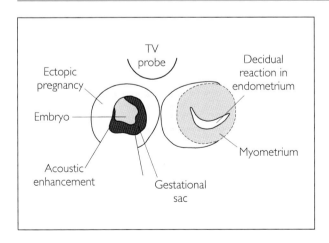

Ectopic pregnancy

Embryo

Acoustic enhancement

TV probe

Gestational sac

Decidual reaction in endometrium

Myometrium

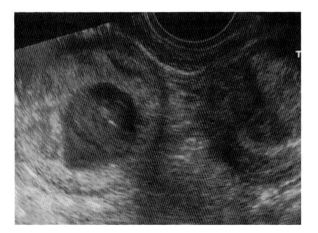

- In reality, it can be difficult to distinguish these adnexal masses from other pathology, e.g. complex ovarian lesions (see the pathology section in the chapter on the female pelvis)

A normal TV scan does not exclude an ectopic pregnancy. Report: An empty uterus is seen. Whilst the pregnancy test is positive, this remains a pregnancy of unknown location. Serial BhCG testing is advised to aid in the future management of this case.

Thyroid

ANATOMY

Transverse section

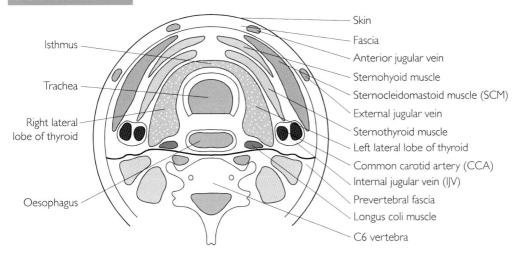

- Isthmus
- Trachea
- Right lateral lobe of thyroid
- Oesophagus
- Skin
- Fascia
- Anterior jugular vein
- Sternohyoid muscle
- Sternocleidomastoid muscle (SCM)
- External jugular vein
- Sternothyroid muscle
- Left lateral lobe of thyroid
- Common carotid artery (CCA)
- Internal jugular vein (IJV)
- Prevertebral fascia
- Longus coli muscle
- C6 vertebra

Anterior view

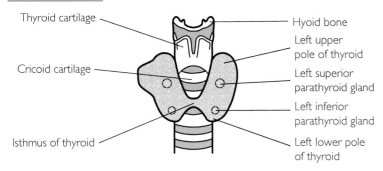

- Thyroid cartilage
- Cricoid cartilage
- Isthmus of thyroid
- Hyoid bone
- Left upper pole of thyroid
- Left superior parathyroid gland
- Left inferior parathyroid gland
- Left lower pole of thyroid

● Key points

1 The thyroid gland has two lateral lobes and a midline isthmus.
2 The lateral lobes are often asymmetrical; the right tends to be more vascular and larger.
3 Each lobe has a superior and inferior pole.
4 The normal craniocaudal length of the thyroid gland is <4 cm.
5 There are four parathyroid glands lying posterior to the thyroid gland.
6 The normal craniocaudal length of each parathyroid gland is <6 mm.

Surface landmarks of thyroid

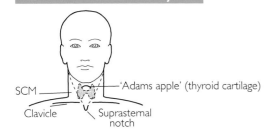

- SCM
- Clavicle
- 'Adams apple' (thyroid cartilage)
- Suprasternal notch

DOI: 10.1201/9781003381655-12

PERFORMING THE SCAN

- **Patient position:** Supine with neck extended.
- **Preparation:** None.
- **Probe:** High-frequency (7.5 MHz) linear.
- **Machine:** Select 'small parts' preset on machine. Use tissue harmonics if the SNR is poor. Use compound imaging and at least two focal points, with one positioned at the posterior aspect of the thyroid gland.
- **Method:** Do not apply any pressure to the probe, as this is uncomfortable for the patient.

PROBE POSITION   INSTRUCTIONS

1 TS

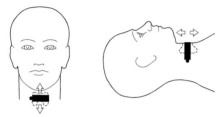

- Place the probe just inferior to the thyroid cartilage.
- Scan through the thyroid in TS.
- The normal thyroid gland:
  - is more echogenic than the SCM
  - has a homogenous echotexture
  - is highly vascular
- Take note of the:
  - echogenicity
  - surface outline
  - texture
  - size
- Check for any:
  - calcification (micro or macro)
  - solid lesions (size, mass effect)
  - cysts
- Depending on the clinical history and ultrasound findings, turn on colour/power Doppler to assess for:
  - hyperaemia
  - neovascularization of any solid lesions
- Take representative image(s).

2 LS

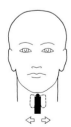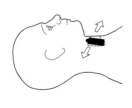

- Rotate the probe clockwise through 90°.
- Scan through the thyroid in LS.
- Observe the thyroid characteristics as described in Step 1.
- If the whole gland is not on the screen, it may be enlarged; measure the craniocaudal length to check for a goitre. If necessary, use a dual screen. The normal craniocaudal thyroid length is <4 cm.
- Take representative image(s).

WHAT TO LOOK FOR

SCAN IMAGE

1

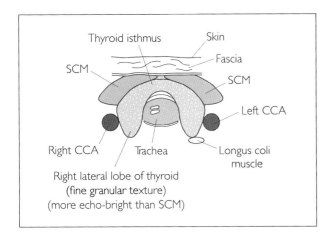

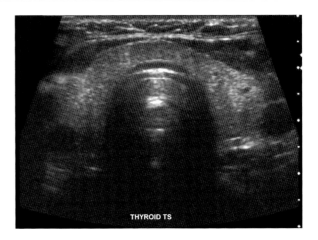

2

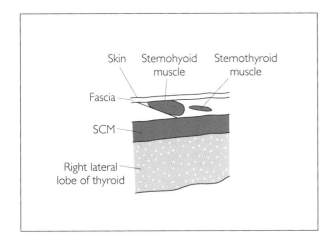

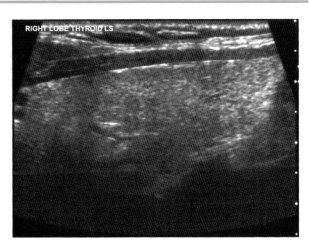

PATHOLOGY

● 1 *Graves' disease*

This is an autoimmune disease with a female-to-male ratio of 8:1 and usually affects ages 20–40 years. This is usually associated with hyperthyroidism.

Ultrasound features
- Diffusely enlarged thyroid
- Homogenous, i.e. loss of fine granular echotexture
- Normal echogenicity or echo-bright
- Displays increased blood flow with colour/power Doppler

● 2 *Hashimoto's thyroiditis*

This is an autoimmune disease with a female-to-male ratio of 12:1 and usually affects ages 30–50 years. Usually hypothyroid.

Ultrasound features
- Diffusely enlarged thyroid
- Heterogeneous, with coarse echotexture
- Echo-poor

● 3 *Multinodular goitre*

This has a female-to-male ratio of 3:1 and usually affects ages 50–70 years. Usually normal thyroid function.

Ultrasound features
- Irregular enlarged thyroid
- Heterogeneous with multiple nodules
- Nodules can be solid, cystic or solid/cystic
- Nodules > 7 mm

WHAT TO LOOK FOR

SCAN IMAGE

1 Graves' disease

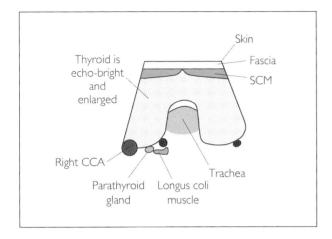

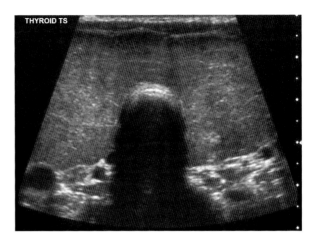

2 Hashimoto's thyroiditis

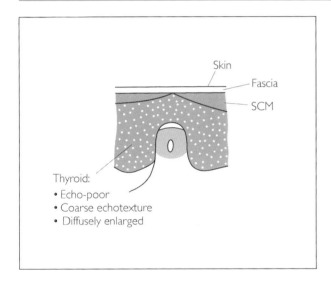

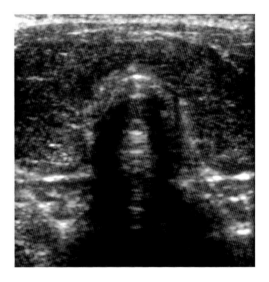

3 Multinodular goitre

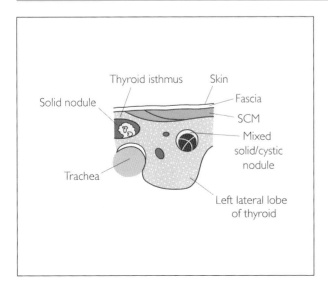

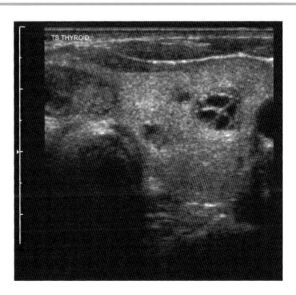

● 4 Thyroid carcinoma

There are five types: papillary, follicular, anaplastic, medullary and lymphoma. The female-to-male ratio is 3:1. Papillary and follicular types affect ages 20–40 years and anaplastic ages >60 years. Note that calcification is useful to determine whether a nodule is malignant or benign:

- microcalcification (<2 mm): high positive predictive value for malignancy
- macrocalcification (>2 mm): degeneration/post-inflammatory, often rim calcifications

Ultrasound features
- Predominantly single, but may be multiple
- Mass usually >7 mm
- Solid or partially cystic
- Irregular margins with breaching of any pseudocapsule that may be present.
- Exert mass effect
- Echo-poor
- Microcalcification
- Hypervascular (with colour/power Doppler)

WHAT TO LOOK FOR **SCAN IMAGE**

4a Thyroid carcinoma

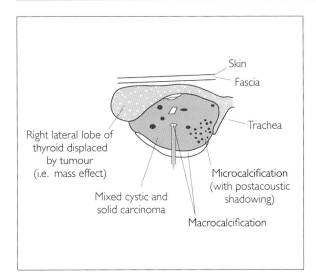

Skin

Fascia

Right lateral lobe of
thyroid displaced
by tumour
(i.e. mass effect)

Trachea

Microcalcification
(with postacoustic
shadowing)

Mixed cystic and
solid carcinoma

Macrocalcification

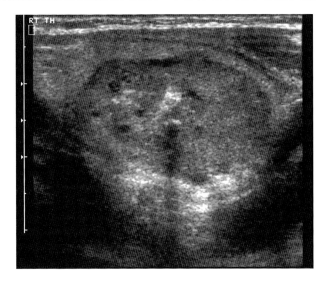

4b Thyroid carcinoma

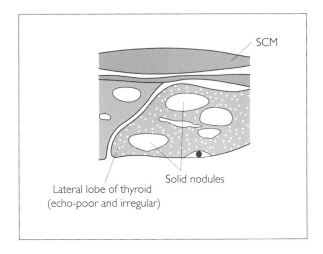

SCM

Lateral lobe of thyroid
(echo-poor and irregular)

Solid nodules

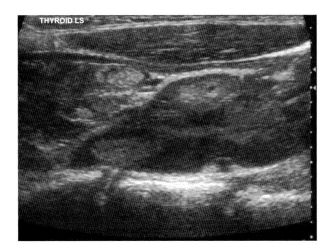

● 5 *Enlarged parathyroid glands*

Causes include adenoma, carcinoma and hyperplasia (e.g. in patients with chronic renal failure).

Ultrasound features

- \>6 mm
- More echo-poor than thyroid
- Hypervascular (with colour/power Doppler)
- Diffusely enlarged (with hyperplasia)
- Heterogeneous (with adenoma or carcinoma)

Hint: Do not confuse the longus coli muscle with an enlarged parathyroid gland. Confirm that it is a parathyroid gland by scanning in TS and LS.

● 6 *Cervical lymphadenopathy*

Causes include infection, metastases and lymphoma.

Ultrasound features of reactive nodes

- Elliptical: Long axis <10 mm, short axis <7 mm
- Echo-bright hilum of fat and echo-poor cortex

Regular branching pattern of vessels from the hilum on colour Doppler.

Ultrasound features of pathological nodes

- Spherical
- 0 mm long axis
- Loss of echo-bright hilum
- Loss of a normal branching vascular pattern with the recruitment of other vessels on colour Doppler.
- May exert a mass effect on surrounding structures

WHAT TO LOOK FOR   **SCAN IMAGE**

5 Enlarged parathyroid gland

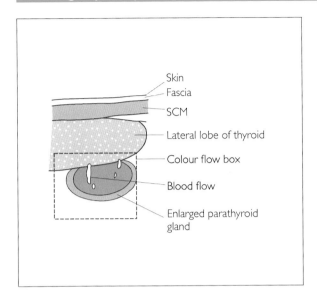

- Skin
- Fascia
- SCM
- Lateral lobe of thyroid
- Colour flow box
- Blood flow
- Enlarged parathyroid gland

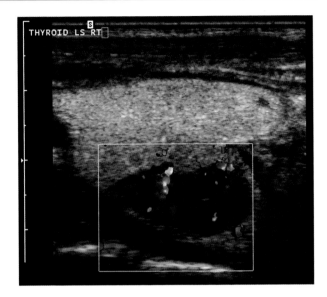

6 Cervical lymphadenopathy

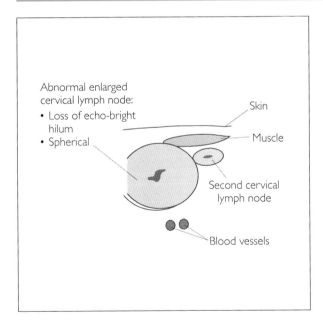

Abnormal enlarged cervical lymph node:
- Loss of echo-bright hilum
- Spherical

- Skin
- Muscle
- Second cervical lymph node
- Blood vessels

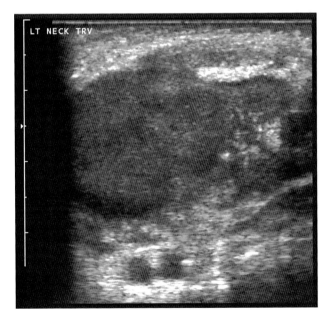

13 Focused assessment with sonography in trauma (FAST)

- A FAST examination is a targeted ultrasound study used to survey major trauma patients.
- The aim is to look for large intraperitoneal free fluid collections that provide indirect evidence of solid organ injury that may require urgent surgical intervention.
- FAST may also be used to look for a pericardial effusion as an indirect sign of cardiac injury.
- It should be noted that ultrasound has a low sensitivity for the detection of solid organ injury; rather, a FAST scan should be regarded as a screening tool and, if positive for free fluid, is usually followed by a multidetector CT examination to pinpoint the exact source of bleeding or laparotomy if the patient is haemodynamically unstable.
- FAST scans are usually performed in the emergency department and often with a portable machine, which can make the scan technically challenging to perform and interpret. For example, lighting conditions are often suboptimal for performing ultrasound and acoustic windows may be limited by patient immobilization and life support/monitoring equipment.
- It will not always be possible to perform the scan in the standard way and the operator must use whatever acoustic windows are available. It is important not to waste too much time trying to acquire good quality images.
- The sensitivity of a FAST scan to detect free fluid depends on the volume of fluid and its distribution, and a negative FAST scan cannot exclude significant visceral injury.

DOI: 10.1201/9781003381655-13

PERFORMING THE SCAN

- **Patient position:** Supine.
- **Preparation:** None.
- **Probe:** Low-frequency (3–5 MHz) curvilinear
- **Machine:** Select the abdominal preset mode. Use tissue harmonics and compound imaging if the SNR is poor or with obese patients.
- **Method:** Scan over the four key areas to identify free fluid and pericardial effusion (see below).
- Although we advise recording images, it is recognized that in many situations no images can be saved and the written report of the operator in the notes is an acceptable record of the examination.

PROBE POSITION

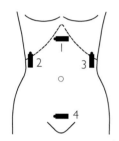

INSTRUCTIONS

1 Substernal
2 RUQ
3 LUQ
4 Pelvis

1 Substernal: TS heart

- Place the probe TS in the upper abdomen in the midline and angle upwards towards the patient's head, i.e. scanning up and under the costal margin.
- Look for the heart chambers with the right ventricle appearing in front of the left ventricle (more towards the top of the screen) and having a more elongated appearance than the left. Adjust the depth and FOV accordingly. Set the focal zone to the middle of the left ventricle.
- Scan through as much of the heart as acoustic windows will allow, paying particular attention to the area around it where a pericardial effusion will be seen if present.
- If a pericardial effusion is present:
  - Measure its maximal thickness perpendicular to the cardiac chamber.
- Acquire representative image(s).

2 Right upper quadrant: LS Morrison's pouch

- Place the probe LS in the RUQ to image the right kidney and right lobe of the liver together.
- It may be necessary to scan along one of the lower intercostal spaces to get a good acoustic window.
- Look for any fluid in the hepatorenal space (Morrison's pouch).
- Acquire representative image(s).

WHAT TO LOOK FOR

SCAN IMAGE

1

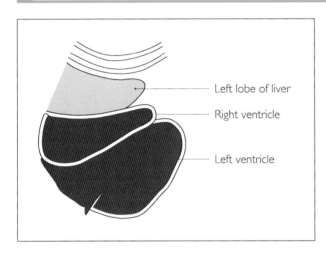

- Left lobe of liver
- Right ventricle
- Left ventricle

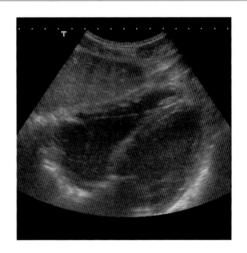

2

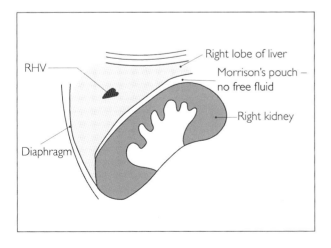

RHV

Right lobe of liver

Morrison's pouch – no free fluid

Right kidney

Diaphragm

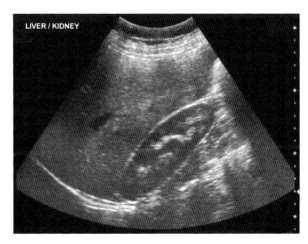

PROBE POSITION   **INSTRUCTIONS**

3 Left upper quadrant: LS splenorenal space

- Place the probe LS in the LUQ to image the left kidney and spleen together.
- It may be necessary to scan along one of the lower intercostal spaces to get a good acoustic window.
- Look for any fluid in the splenorenal space.
- Acquire representative image(s).

4 TS pelvis

- Place the probe midline in the suprapubic area.
- Look for the bladder (may be largely collapsed) and adjust the depth and FOV to target the area immediately behind the bladder.
- In females, the uterus lies posterior to the bladder and it is the rectouterine pouch that needs to be assessed (pouch of Douglas).
- Look for any fluid in the pouch of Douglas (females) or rectovesical pouch (males).
- A small amount of fluid in the pouch of Douglas can be a normal appearance in a female of child-bearing age, depending upon the stage of the menstrual cycle.
- Acquire representative image(s).

WHAT TO LOOK FOR

SCAN IMAGE

3

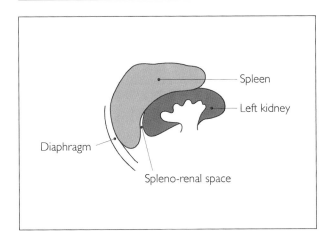

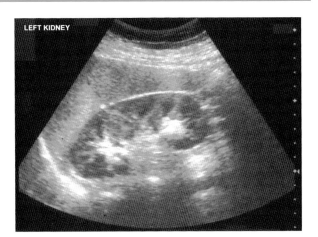

4

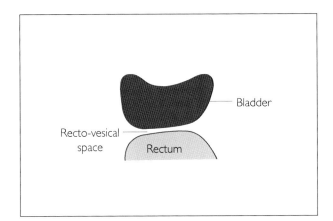

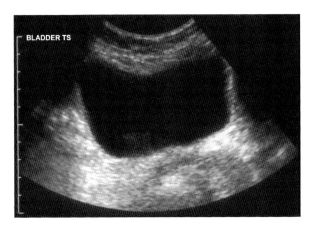

PATHOLOGY

● 1 *Pericardial effusion*

This is an accumulation of fluid within the pericardial space that can impair cardiac function by compressive effects on the cardiac chambers. A pericardial effusion with clinical signs of cardiac tamponade (a rise in jugular venous pressure on inspiration) requires urgent drainage (pericardiocentesis) to alleviate symptoms. A pericardial effusion can be graded according to its depth, although it should be noted that a small effusion that has developed rapidly often produces more symptoms than a large effusion that has developed slowly due to adaptive stretching of the pericardial sac.

Ultrasound features
- Echo-free fluid collection within the pericardial space
- Depth of fluid grading system:
  - Small: maximal depth < 1 cm
  - Moderate: maximal depth 1–2 cm
  - Large: maximal depth > 2 cm
- Features that suggest cardiac tamponade are collapse of the right atrial and ventricular free wall in the diastolic phase of the cardiac cycle

● 2 *Abdomen–pelvic free fluid*

Fluid tends to accumulate in predictable locations within the abdomen (flanks) and pelvis (rectovesical pouch/ pouch of Douglas) when the patient is in the supine position. It appears as an echo-free collection without defined margins. Free fluid can be caused by a wide range of pathological conditions, including trauma with visceral organ or bowel injury, liver cirrhosis, renal failure and right heart failure. It can also be seen as a normal finding in patients being treated with peritoneal dialysis. Although the commonest cause for free fluid in the major trauma setting will be intraperitoneal haemorrhage secondary to visceral organ injury, alternative causes should still be borne in mind.

Ultrasound features
- Echo-free collection within the hepatorenal space, splenorenal space or pelvis

WHAT TO LOOK FOR

SCAN IMAGE

1 Pericardial effusion

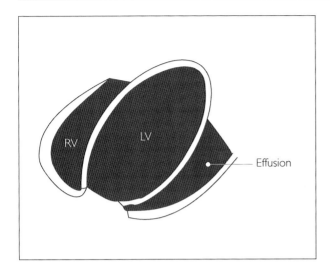

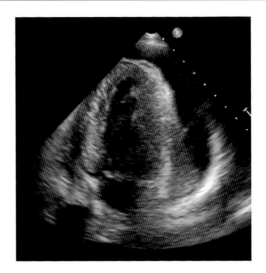

2 Abdomen–pelvic free fluid

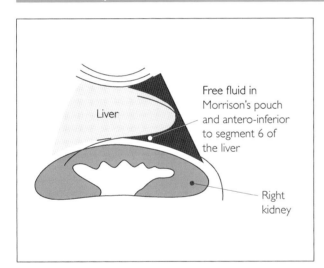

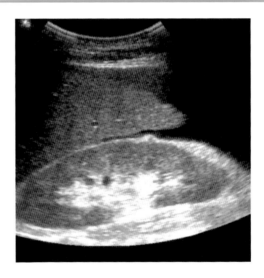

And/or

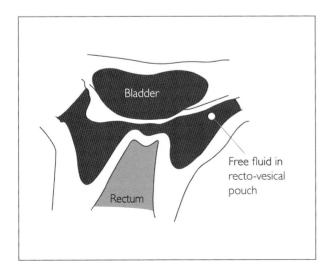

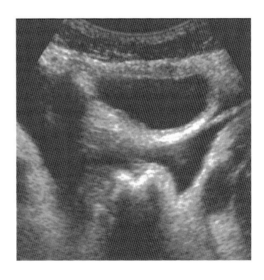

14 *Breast*

ANATOMY

- Normal breasts vary widely in their composition of fatty and glandular tissue.
- Fine echo-bright (Coopers) ligaments run through the breast, dividing it into lobules.
- Deep structures including the chest wall musculature and ribs appear echo-poor but should be routinely assessed.
- Normal glandular tissue is of intermediate echogenicity and can contain hypoechoic lymph nodes.
- Glandular tissue in lactating women demonstrates hypertrophied glandular components.

Sagittal section through breast and anatomy of normal breast

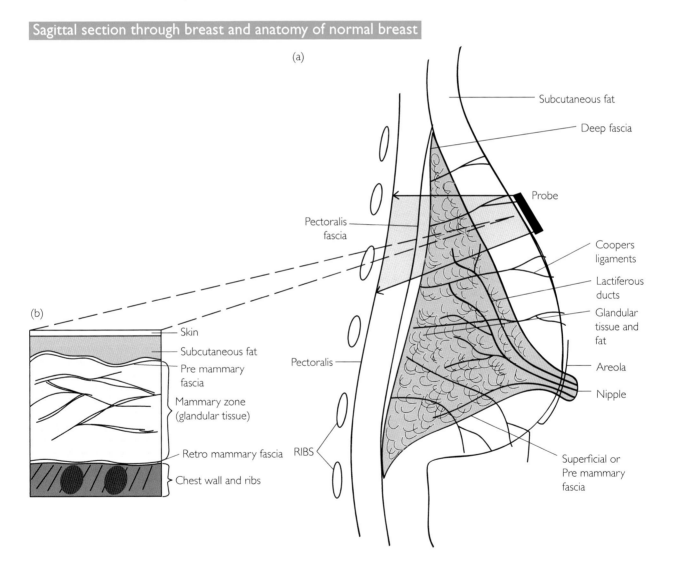

(a)

Subcutaneous fat

Deep fascia

Probe

Coopers ligaments

Lactiferous ducts

Glandular tissue and fat

Areola

Nipple

Superficial or Pre mammary fascia

Pectoralis fascia

Pectoralis

RIBS

(b)

Skin

Subcutaneous fat

Pre mammary fascia

Mammary zone (glandular tissue)

Retro mammary fascia

Chest wall and ribs

DOI: 10.1201/9781003381655-14

PERFORMING THE SCAN

- **Patient position:** Supine with ipsilateral arm abducted, elbow flexed, hand cupped behind the head.
  - to assess the outer quadrants, the patient may need to assume a posterior oblique posture
  - use a wedge or cushion back support to elevate the scanned breast by 30°–45°
  - obliquity depends on breast size, pendulousness and location of lesion
  - aim to spread breast tissue evenly to maximize resolution

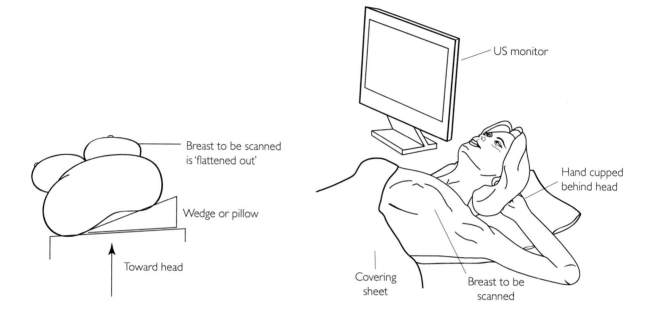

Breast to be scanned is 'flattened out'

Wedge or pillow

Toward head

US monitor

Hand cupped behind head

Covering sheet

Breast to be scanned

- **Preparation:**
  - It is advised that a chaperone (e.g. breast care nurse) be present during the examination.
  - Confirm patient details, explain the nature of the examination and take verbal consent.
  - Operator stands on the patient's right-hand side, US machine to the upper left of table, regardless of which breast is to be examined.

> **Have the most recent mammograms available to guide examination and US**

  - Patient bra removed and gown open at front.
  - Expose the breast and axilla (keep the other breast covered).
  - Palpate the lesion between the index and middle finger.

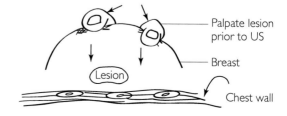

Palpate lesion prior to US

Breast

Lesion

Chest wall

- **Probe:** High-frequency 7.5–12 MHz linear probe penetrates most breasts.
- **Machine:** Select small parts/breast preset mode.
- **Method:** Start with a targeted scan in the quadrant where the palpable lump/abnormality is indicated by the breast physician or surgeon.
  - if there is no palpable abnormality, start scanning in the quadrant where mammographic abnormality is suspected
  - confirm the side and site of abnormality with the patient
  - scan the entire breast only if multifocal abnormalities are evident on the targeted US
  - scan the **IPSILATERAL** axilla if malignancy is suspected
  - scan slowly in anti-radial/radial planes and LS/TS using an **OVERLAPPING** scan strip technique

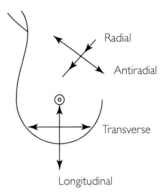

  - acquire more than one representative image in two or more planes if pathology found
  - annotate using laterality (R/L), breast quadrant and breast icon, if available
    'Clockface' annotation and distance from the nipple are useful adjuncts
  - Adopt your local breast department protocol

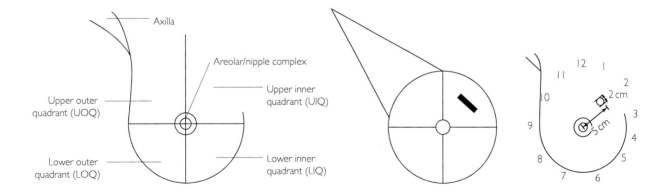

● *Tips*

- Use a thick layer of gel when assessing a near field or superficial lesion.
- Use pressure, additional gel, or a **gel stand-off technique*** to visualize the nipple.
- Oblique angling of the probe around the nipple helps show tissues deep to the nipple.
- In larger breasts, a mid or lower frequency range transducer may be required to gain adequate penetration.
- Ensure that there is OVERLAP between passes, over the borders of the breast and into adjacent quadrants with the US beam, to reduce the risk of missed lesions.
- Mark the skin with a plastic needle cap or ballpoint pen at the heel of the probe, to guide biopsy approach.

> ***** Stand off technique refers to using a layer of thick US gel and minimal transducer pressure to visualize a near field or retro-areola lesion.

WHAT TO LOOK FOR   SCAN IMAGE

1 Normal breast TS

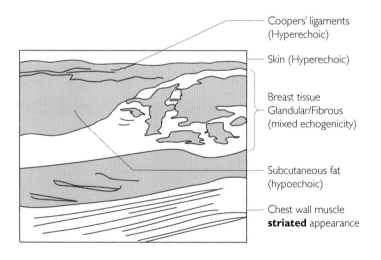

Coopers' ligaments (Hyperechoic)

Skin (Hyperechoic)

Breast tissue Glandular/Fibrous (mixed echogenicity)

Subcutaneous fat (hypoechoic)

Chest wall muscle **striated** appearance

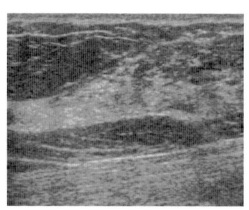

WHAT TO LOOK FOR   **SCAN IMAGE**

2 Normal lactating breast TS

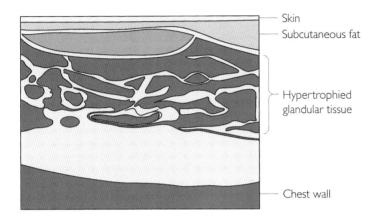
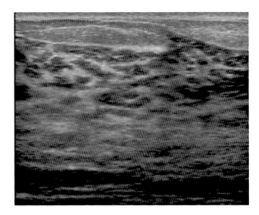

— Skin
— Subcutaneous fat

— Hypertrophied glandular tissue

— Chest wall

3 Normal axilla

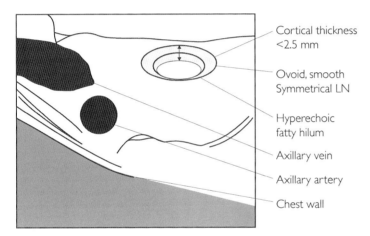
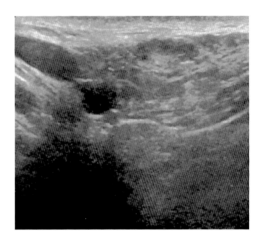

— Cortical thickness <2.5 mm

— Ovoid, smooth Symmetrical LN

— Hyperechoic fatty hilum

— Axillary vein

— Axillary artery

— Chest wall

PATHOLOGY

The primary aims of breast US are:

- to make a more specific diagnosis in patients with **clinical or mammographic abnormality**
- to confirm the presence and extent of malignant disease
- to guide and expedite intervention e.g. biopsy or cyst drainage
- common findings include simple or complex cystic lesions, solid malignant lesions with or without axillary lymph node abnormality and benign solid lesions

> US characterization of clinically palpable or mammographically evident breast mass should take place as part of a **'triple assessment'** at a designated outpatient clinic (e.g. 'breast symptomatic' clinic or 'screening assessment' clinic); where clinical, mammographic and ultrasound evaluation can be carried out concurrently with nursing and clinical support.

The following descriptive terms are used:

- **Shape:** round, lobular, irregular.
- **Margin:** well-defined, ill-defined.
- **Density:** fat equivalent, hypodense (but not fat equivalent), isodense to parenchyma, hyperdense.
- **Lesion axis:** taller than wide, perpendicular to skin or parallel to skin.
- **Echoes:** anechoic (cysts), hypoechoic, isoechoic or hyperechoic relative to the breast.
- **Posterior acoustic change:** enhancement, shadowing or none.
- **Mobility:** good or immobile.
- **Surrounding structures:** intact, displaced, distorted (e.g. by scar or carcinoma).
- **Compressibility:** good, none.
- **Presence of microcalcification:** yes/no.
- **Axillary lymph nodes:** abnormal/normal.

> **Standard US scoring criteria for breast pathology:**
> **U1** = Normal
> **U2** = Benign
> **U3** = Indeterminate/Probably benign
> **U4** = Probably malignant
> **U5** = Definitely malignant

1 Solid malignant breast lesions

Malignant features
- Spiculation
- Thick echogenic halo
- Microlobulation (1–2 mm)
- Complete or partial acoustic shadowing
- 'Taller-than-wide' vertical orientation
- Angular margins
- Intraductal extension
- Microcalcification
- Hypoechogenicity
- Non-compressible
- Distorted surrounding tissues

- Incidence of cancer increases with age; majority in over 50 age group.
- Most common presentation is a painless lump.
- Many histopathological entities exist (e.g. low to high grade, ductal, lobular, tubular, colloid, papillary, etc.) with variable US appearance.
- Ultrasound differentiation is based on the presence of multiple features, which if combined, have high sensitivity for malignancy.

WHAT TO LOOK FOR

SCAN IMAGE

Solid malignant lesions scoring U4 or U5

1a

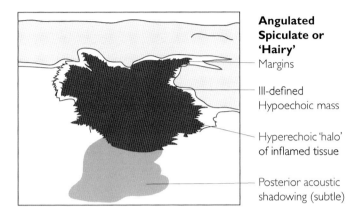

Angulated Spiculate or 'Hairy'
Margins

Ill-defined Hypoechoic mass

Hyperechoic 'halo' of inflamed tissue

Posterior acoustic shadowing (subtle)

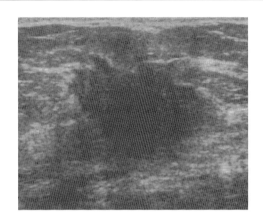

1b

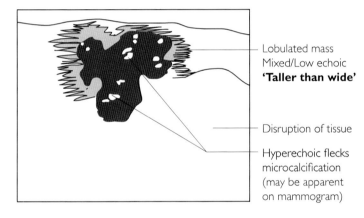

Lobulated mass Mixed/Low echoic **'Taller than wide'**

Disruption of tissue

Hyperechoic flecks microcalcification (may be apparent on mammogram)

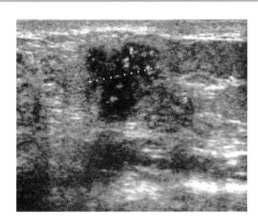

1c

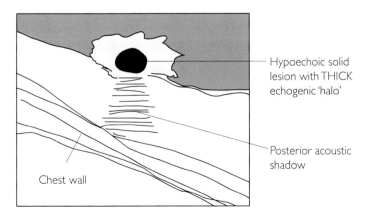

Hypoechoic solid lesion with THICK echogenic 'halo'

Posterior acoustic shadow

Chest wall

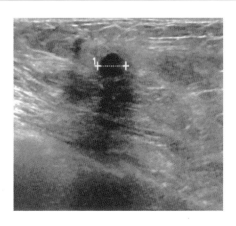

WHAT TO LOOK FOR   **SCAN IMAGE**

1d

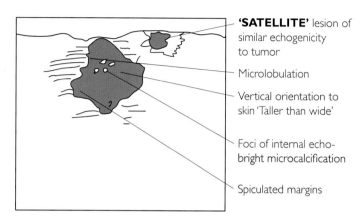

'**SATELLITE**' lesion of similar echogenicity to tumor

Microlobulation

Vertical orientation to skin 'Taller than wide'

Foci of internal echo-bright microcalcification

Spiculated margins

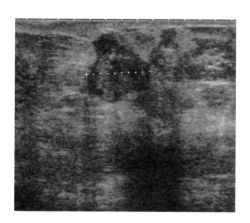

1e

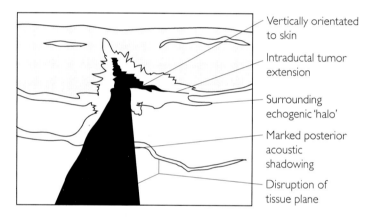

Vertically orientated to skin

Intraductal tumor extension

Surrounding echogenic 'halo'

Marked posterior acoustic shadowing

Disruption of tissue plane

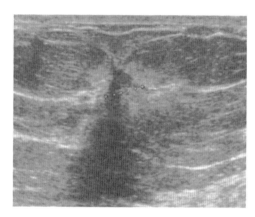

1f

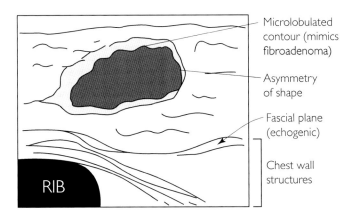

Microlobulated contour (mimics fibroadenoma)

Asymmetry of shape

Fascial plane (echogenic)

Chest wall structures

RIB

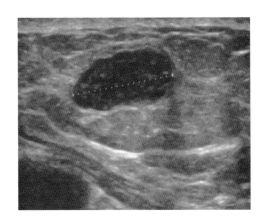

COMMON BENIGN MIMICS OF BREAST CANCER

1 Diabetic mastopathy

- Usually presenting as a hard lump in pre-menopausal diabetics
- Non-specific mammographic findings
- Often exhibits malignant ultrasound features similar to invasive carcinoma, resulting in biopsy

2 Fat necrosis

- Under half accompanied by history of localized trauma (e.g. seat belt, pets, sport) or breast surgery
- Spectrum of US appearances due to degree of inflammatory tissue response
- Biopsy if not 'typical' (i.e. hyper-reflective)
- May appear as:
  - focus of increased echogenicity of subcutaneous tissue is most typical
  - irregular, solid, anechoic mass with posterior enhancement
  - complex cyst with internal echo or nodule

'Be careful': Radial scar
- Hypoechoic lesion mimicking breast cancer following breast surgery
- Best assessed by mammography
- Occurs typically within 5 years of breast surgery
- Ultrasound findings non-specific therefore US has LIMITED role
- Often results in biopsy

WHAT TO LOOK FOR

SCAN IMAGE

1 Diabetic mastopathy

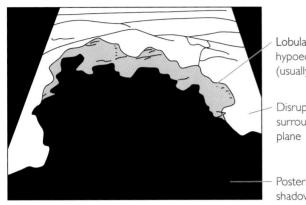

Lobulated ill-defined hypoechoic area (usually large)

Disruption of surrounding tissue plane

Posterior acoustic shadowing

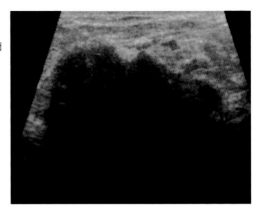

2a Fat necrosis (typical)

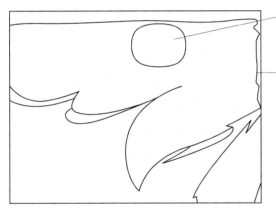

Focus of increased reflectivity

Subcutaneous fat of relativity low echogenicity

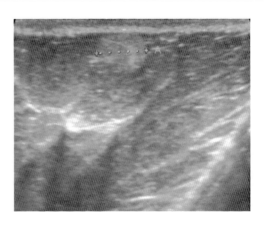

2b Fat necrosis (atypical)

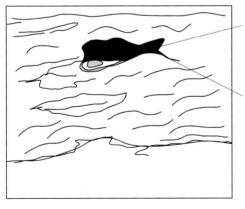

Ill-defined focus of mixed echogenicity within subcutaneous fat

'Wider than tall'

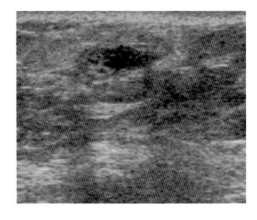

SOLID BENIGN LESIONS

Solid lesions without malignant features should be assessed for benign features:

- Purely hyper-echoic tissue
- Ovoid, wider-than-tall shape
- Gently lobulated
- Complete thin echogenic capsule

1 Fibroadenoma

- More common in the young; oestrogen is a factor in growth; involution after menopause
- Usually elliptical, gently lobulated and iso/mildly hypoechoic to fat
- Classically have a pseudocapsule of compressed tissue
- Invariably 'wider than tall'; Normally <3 cm in size
- May grow rapidly (e.g. during pregnancy) and become giant FA (6–10 cm)
- May be multiple and bilateral
- Usually mobile and mildly compressible with probe
- May undergo sclerosis, hyalinization or calcification, (1:1000 undergo malignant change)
- Confirmation biopsy is usually performed in women >35 years

2 Lipoma

- Benign overgrowth of adipose tissue; well-defined, slow growing
- May contain glandular or capillary tissue
- Isoechoic or hypoechoic to surrounding fat
- May have internal echogenic septae parallel to the skin
- Demonstrates decreasing AP diameter with mild transducer pressure
- Usually in subcutaneous fat layer or axillary fat

WHAT TO LOOK FOR

SCAN IMAGE

1a Fibroadenoma

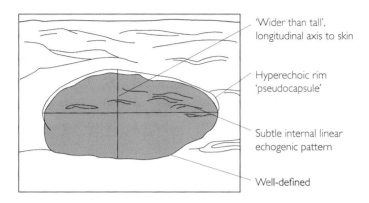

'Wider than tall', longitudinal axis to skin

Hyperechoic rim 'pseudocapsule'

Subtle internal linear echogenic pattern

Well-defined

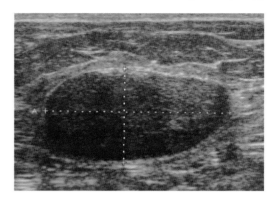

1b Fibroadenoma

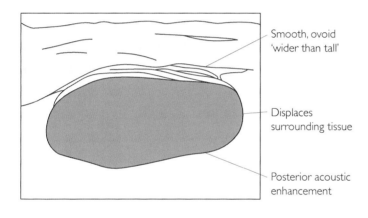

Smooth, ovoid 'wider than tall'

Displaces surrounding tissue

Posterior acoustic enhancement

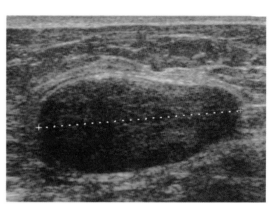

2 Lipoma

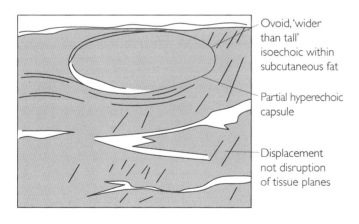

Ovoid, 'wider than tall' isoechoic within subcutaneous fat

Partial hyperechoic capsule

Displacement not disruption of tissue planes

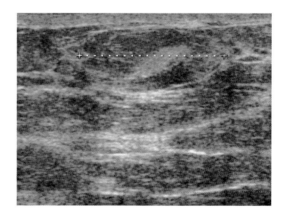

3 Intramammary lymph node

- Elliptical, hypoechoic, <10 mm, cortical thickness <2.5 mm
- Usually lie in upper outer quadrants or axillary 'tail'
- Doppler will demonstrate flow within the echogenic hilus; this confirms diagnosis

4 Epidermoid inclusion cyst (or sebaceous cyst)

- Typically located at inferior or medial breast margins (near bra wire)
- Small, hypoechoic, located within skin or close to skin surface
- If within skin: 'claw sign' of hyperechoic skin surrounds lesion
- Associated 'track' extending to skin surface may be visible
- TIP: use 'stand-off ' gel technique to demonstrate lesion in near field

WHAT TO LOOK FOR

SCAN IMAGE

3 Intramammary lymph node

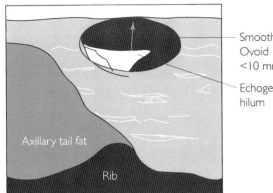

- Smooth
  Ovoid
  <10 mm TS diameter

- Echogenic
  hilum

Axillary tail fat

Rib

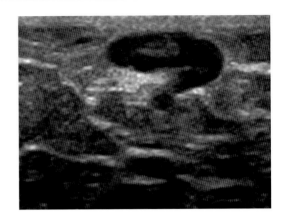

4 Epidermoid inclusion cyst

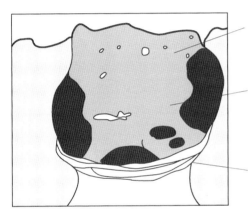

- Superficial location
  within or involving
  skin ± 'crab claw' sign

- Mixed cystic/solid
  echogenicity
  with hyperechoic
  fragments (debris)

- Posterior acoustic
  enhancement

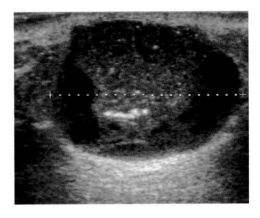

CYSTIC LESIONS

- Classically present as lump(s), nodularity or breast pain
- Hormone dependent with sensitivity to menstrual cycle
- Frequently rupture, atrophy or disappear
- Commonest in upper outer quadrant
- May be simple or complex

1 Simple cysts

- Complete anechoic area
- Well circumscribed with thin echogenic capsule
- Enhanced through transmission
- May be clustered
- May have thin avascular septations or internal debris
- May have punctuate wall calcification
- Do not require biopsy
- Drainage usual if > 1 cm and patient symptomatic – obtain consent

2 Complex cysts

Exhibit US features of inflammatory change:
- Rarely undergo malignant transformation
- Internal debris (pus/haemorrhage)
- Fluid/fluid levels
- Circumferential wall thickening or capsular vascularity
- Mural nodules
- Thick vascular septations or stalk
- Drainage with cytology is usually performed if any solid component present

WHAT TO LOOK FOR   **SCAN IMAGE**

1a Simple cyst

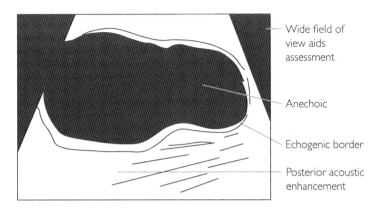

— Wide field of view aids assessment

— Anechoic

— Echogenic border

— Posterior acoustic enhancement

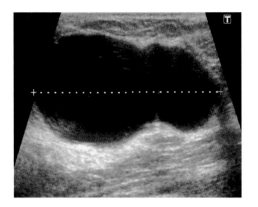

1b Simple cyst

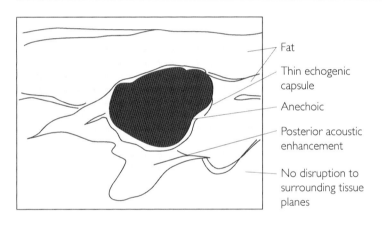

— Fat

— Thin echogenic capsule

— Anechoic

— Posterior acoustic enhancement

— No disruption to surrounding tissue planes

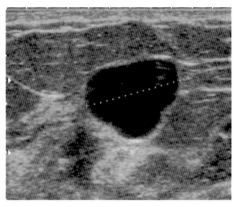

2a

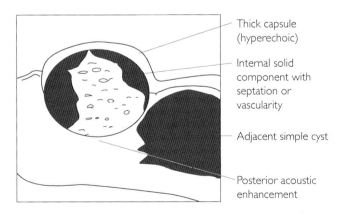

— Thick capsule (hyperechoic)

— Internal solid component with septation or vascularity

— Adjacent simple cyst

— Posterior acoustic enhancement

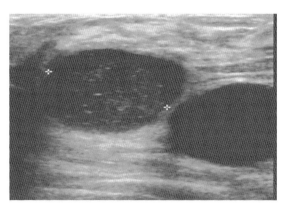

OTHER BENIGN CYSTIC LESIONS

1 Breast abscess

- Usually in diabetic, immunocompromised women
- Frequently a complication of mastitis/galactocele or infected cyst
- Acute onset with local inflammatory changes present
- Echogenic thickening of subcutaneous fat due to oedema
- Subareolar duct dilatation may be associated
- Ultrasound obtains fluid for microbiology and is a method of choice for drainage

WHAT TO LOOK FOR

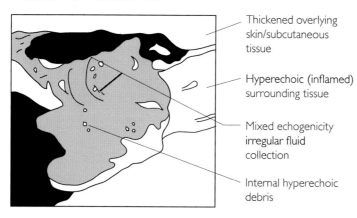

Thickened overlying skin/subcutaneous tissue

Hyperechoic (inflamed) surrounding tissue

Mixed echogenicity irregular fluid collection

Internal hyperechoic debris

SCAN IMAGE

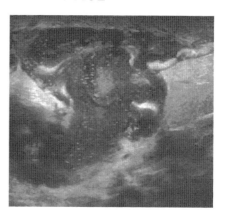

2 Galactocele

- Essentially same appearance as breast abscess
- Painless lump in breastfeeding mothers
- Contain emulsified fat droplets so appear anechoic
- Peripheral and multilocular or central and unilocular
- Low level internal echoes or fat/fluid level
- Aspiration diagnostic and therapeutic

3 Mastitis

- Often associated with abscess or galactocele
- Echogenic thickening of subcutaneous fat due to oedema
- Epidermis > 3 mm thick

WHAT TO LOOK FOR

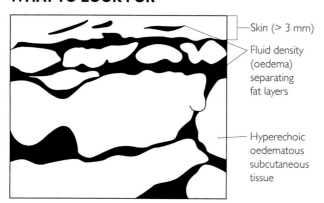

Skin (> 3 mm)

Fluid density (oedema) separating fat layers

Hyperechoic oedematous subcutaneous tissue

SCAN IMAGE

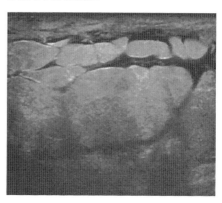

DUCT ECTASIA

- Dilated breast ducts >3 mm AP on US
- More common in middle-aged smokers
- Usually in retroareolar region
- Cause of non-cyclical breast pain or nipple discharge

WHAT TO LOOK FOR

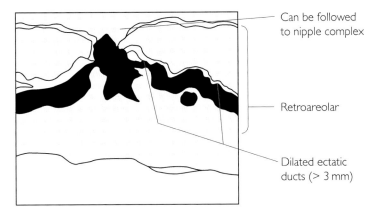

Can be followed to nipple complex

Retroareolar

Dilated ectatic ducts (> 3 mm)

SCAN IMAGE

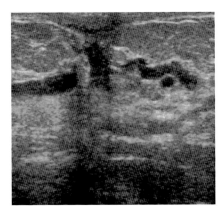

SOLITARY INTRADUCTAL PAPILLOMA

- Well-defined, solid, smooth hypoechoic lesion in a dilated/cystic duct
- Broad-based or peduncular with vascularity
- More common in peri/postmenopausal women
- Solitary lesions are invariably benign
- N.B. Multiple papillomas carry a seven times increased risk of breast carcinoma
- Warning sign – bloody nipple discharge

WHAT TO LOOK FOR

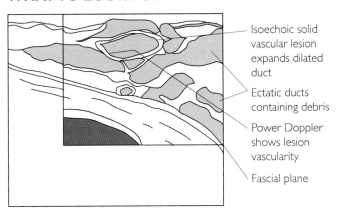

Isoechoic solid vascular lesion expands dilated duct

Ectatic ducts containing debris

Power Doppler shows lesion vascularity

Fascial plane

SCAN IMAGE

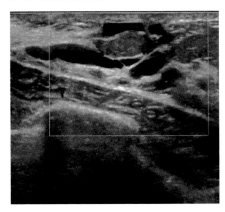

HAEMATOMA/SEROMA

- Post-surgical/post-trauma hypoechoic collection that may contain septae
- Drainage or interval US follow-up is usual
- Use a 14 G needle for guided drainage if fluid is viscous

WHAT TO LOOK FOR

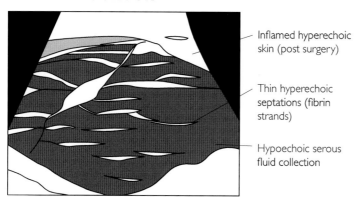

— Inflamed hyperechoic skin (post surgery)

— Thin hyperechoic septations (fibrin strands)

— Hypoechoic serous fluid collection

SCAN IMAGE

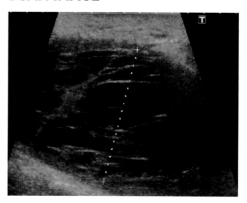

FIBROCYSTIC BREAST DISEASE

- Common cause of breast pain in women over 30, related to hormonal variation
- Spectrum of non-specific findings: microcysts, heterogeneous echogenicity, indeterminate small masses

BE AWARE: May make diagnosis of small cancer more difficult so correlation with mammogram is essential.

WHAT TO LOOK FOR

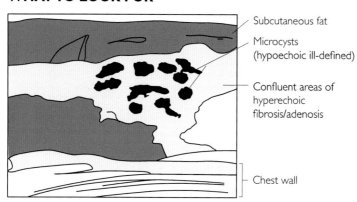

— Subcutaneous fat

— Microcysts (hypoechoic ill-defined)

— Confluent areas of hyperechoic fibrosis/adenosis

— Chest wall

SCAN IMAGE

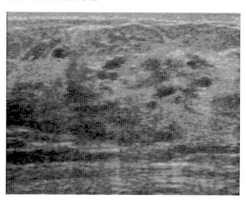

BREAST IMPLANTS

- Mostly silicone, usually in younger or postmastectomy patients
- Hyperechoic capsule should be smooth, not 'ruched'
- Break in capsule indicates rupture
- Reactive enlarged hyperechoic axillary lymph nodes may be present if silicone has leaked

WHAT TO LOOK FOR

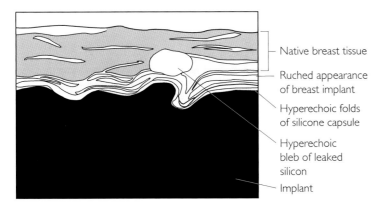

— Native breast tissue

— Ruched appearance of breast implant

— Hyperechoic folds of silicone capsule

— Hyperechoic bleb of leaked silicon

— Implant

SCAN IMAGE

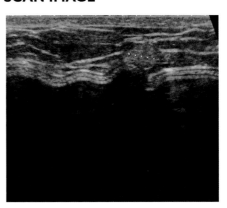

AXILLARY PATHOLOGY

- Any suspicious breast lesion, U3 or above, should prompt a routine ultrasound of ipsilateral axilla.

US criteria for lymph node abnormality

- Asymmetric shape
- Loss of fatty hilum
- Focal enlargement
- Irregular contour
- Cortical thickness >2.3 mm in TS

WHAT TO LOOK FOR

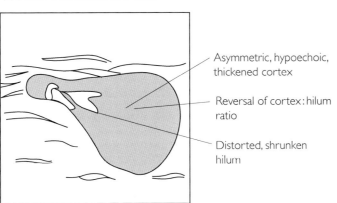

— Asymmetric, hypoechoic, thickened cortex

— Reversal of cortex:hilum ratio

— Distorted, shrunken hilum

SCAN IMAGE

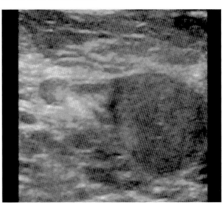

● *Tips*

- Use colour Doppler to locate axillary vessels and lymph node hila
- Switch to small foot plate/MSK probe for needle aspiration or biopsy if access is difficult
- Scan with patient's arm down to better visualize apex of axilla

15 Musculoskeletal

Ultrasound has become an essential technique in musculoskeletal (MSK) imaging. Imaging resolution has significantly improved over the years, with the availability of higher frequency probes making it the first-line investigative tool for a number of musculoskeletal problems. It allows for a dynamic examination and the opportunity to perform diagnostic and therapeutic intervention. Musculoskeletal ultrasound requires a good understanding of the anatomy of the appendicular region as with scanning of any other part of the body.

SHOULDER

This is the most common musculoskeletal ultrasound examination performed.

Common indications for shoulder ultrasound examination are as follows:

- Rotator cuff disease
- Subacromial bursitis and impingement
- Acromioclavicular (AC) joint arthropathy
- Long head biceps disruption

If internal joint derangement is suspected on history and clinical examination, then MRI is the examination of choice.

USEFUL SHOULDER ANATOMY

● Rotator cuff

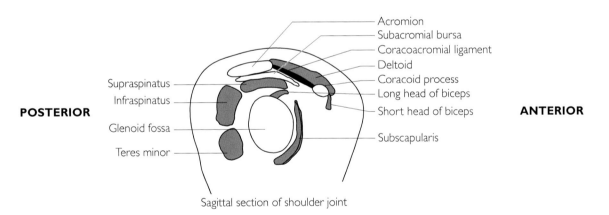

Sagittal section of shoulder joint

The rotator cuff is formed by fusion of four tendons consisting of the supraspinatus, infraspinatus, teres minor, and subscapularis. It overlies the anterior, superior, and posterior aspects of the shoulder. Apart from the subscapularis, which inserts on the lesser tuberosity anteriorly, the remainder of the cuff muscles inserts on the greater tuberosity.

● Long head biceps tendon

Its origin is from the supraglenoid tubercle of scapula and superior glenoid labrum and the tendon courses intraarticularly entering the bicipital sulcus.

DOI: 10.1201/9781003381655-15

PERFORMING THE SCAN
● *Shoulder*

- **Patient position:** Sitting.
- **Preparation:** None.
- **Probe:** High frequency (6–17 MHz) linear.
- **Machine:** Most machines have dedicated shoulder setting. If not, then select MSK. Use the highest frequency, compound imaging and multiple focal zones to improve image quality.
- **Method:** Take a brief history from the patient before commencing the examination. Acquire images systematically covering as described below.

PROBE POSITION	INSTRUCTIONS

1 Long head biceps (LHB) tendon

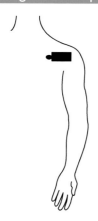

- Hand of the side to be examined is kept over the ipsilateral knee with palm facing upwards.
- Place the probe transversely over the anterior shoulder to locate the bicipital groove, which is seen as a smooth defect. Within the groove, the long head biceps tendon is identified as a smooth, rounded, well-defined structure. Its echogenicity can vary depending on the angle of the probe to the tendon and will be hyperechoic if these are perpendicular to each other.
- Next, turn the probe longitudinally to see the length of the tendon right from its entry into the sulcus to the myotendinous region. Pressure along the caudal aspect of the probe can help straighten the tendon and help visualize it better.
- Examine the tendon for:
  - location
  - integrity
  - thickening and neovascularity
  - tendon sheath effusion and synovitis

2 Subscapularis tendon

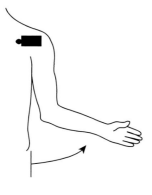

- Place the elbow next to the chest with the forearm parallel to the thigh and externally rotate the forearm.
- Place the probe transversely over the anterior shoulder.
- The subscapularis tendon is recognized as inserting on the medial aspect of bicipital sulcus.
- The probe can be turned in the longitudinal plane, which demonstrates its multipennate structure in the sagittal plane. The tendon can be traced to its insertion.
- Examine the tendon for:
  - integrity
  - any medial subluxation of the long head biceps tendon during the dynamic examination of external rotation

WHAT TO LOOK FOR

SCAN IMAGE

1a

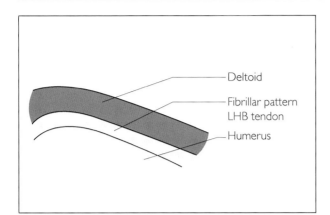

- Deltoid
- Fibrillar pattern
  LHB tendon
- Humerus

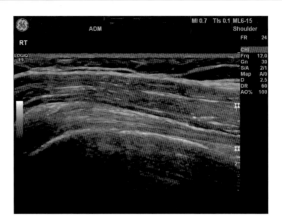

1b

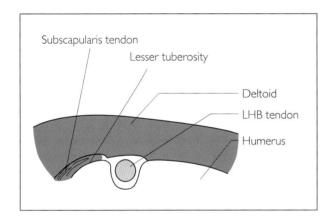

- Subscapularis tendon
- Lesser tuberosity
- Deltoid
- LHB tendon
- Humerus

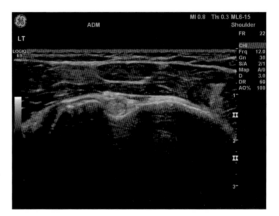

2

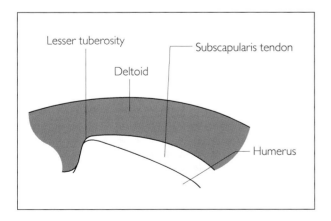

- Lesser tuberosity
- Subscapularis tendon
- Deltoid
- Humerus

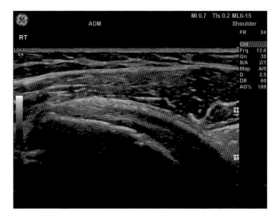

PROBE POSITION

INSTRUCTIONS

3 Supraspinatus and infraspinatus tendons

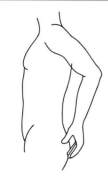

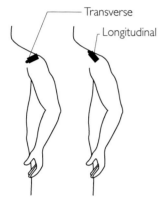

Transverse

Longitudinal

- Ask the patient to place the hand over the ipsilateral back pocket or the lower back/hip region with the palm facing anteriorly.
- Try to keep the elbow in the sagittal plane rather than keeping it outwards.
- Most patients are able to achieve this position. But in cases where this is difficult the following could be tried:
  - pushing the elbow backwards in sagittal plane without attempting to put it over the back pocket or lower back
  - hanging the arm by the side of the patient and internally rotating the hand
- Place the probe in the transverse plane over the anterior shoulder such that the coracoid process is visualized at the margin of the image. Lateral to this is the intra-articular long head biceps (LHB) tendon visualized as a rounded, well-defined hyperechoic structure. The free or the anterior leading edge of the supraspinatus tendon lies immediately lateral to the LHB tendon. The probe is then moved further laterally in the transverse plane to visualize the mid and posterior aspects of the rotator cuff. Subsequently, the cuff is examined in the longitudinal plane with the probe turned in the coronal plane.
- Examine the tendon for:
  - tendinopathic changes
  - tear
  - calcification

4 Subacromial bursa

- Subacromial bursa was examined at the same position as for supraspinatus and infraspinatus tendons (i.e. as 3 above). See 3a and 3b opposite.
- This is a thin bursa overlying the rotator cuff formed by the supraspinatus, infraspinatus and teres minor tendons. It appears as a thin echo-poor layer of fluid between two echo-bright layers of peribursal fat.
- It is examined at the same time as examining the supraspinatus and infraspinatus tendons.
- Examine for:
  - bursal thickening
  - bursal effusion
  - synovitis

WHAT TO LOOK FOR   **SCAN IMAGE**

3a Transverse section

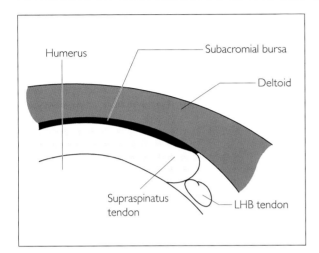

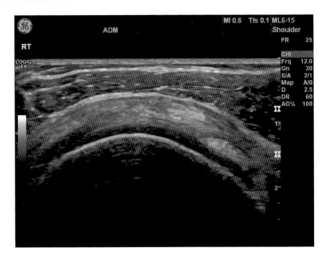

3b Longitudinal section

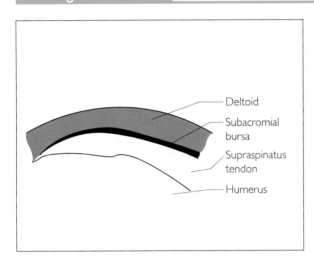

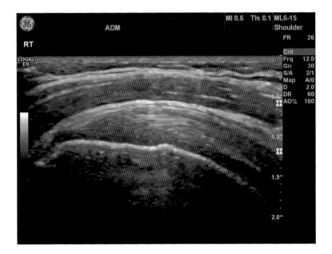

PROBE POSITION	**INSTRUCTIONS**

5 Acromioclavicular joint

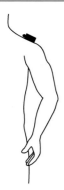

- Place the probe in the coronal plane over the superior shoulder in line with the distal clavicle.
- Dynamic examination can be performed by asking the patient to put the ipsilateral hand over onto the contralateral shoulder.
- Look for:
  - thickening of the joint capsule
  - a gap at the joint
  - osteophytosis
  - joint effusion
  - cyst formation

6 Subacromial impingement

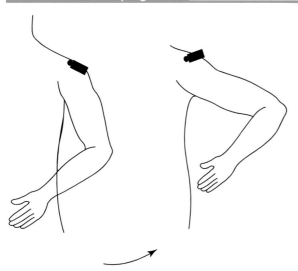

- Keep the probe in the plane of the coracoacromial ligament, which extends from the coracoid process anteriorly to the acromion posteriorly. Subsequently, turn the probe 90° and ask the patient to abduct the shoulder to 90°. In other words, keep the forearm in the sagittal plane at 90° at the elbow joint and then abduct the elbow as far away from the body as possible.
- Examine for any fluid displacement from the subacromial position or bunching of the bursa against the coracoacromial ligament or lateral margin of acromion.

WHAT TO LOOK FOR

SCAN IMAGE

5

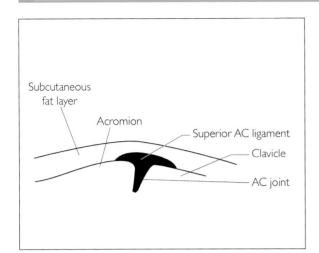

- Subcutaneous fat layer
- Acromion
- Superior AC ligament
- Clavicle
- AC joint

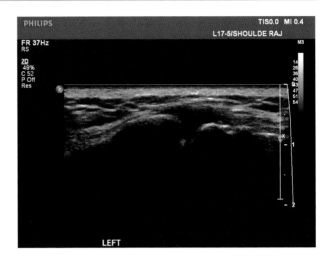

6

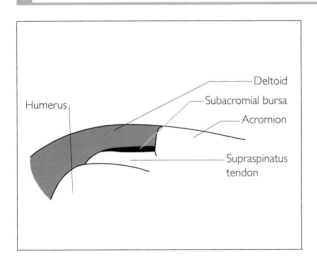

- Humerus
- Deltoid
- Subacromial bursa
- Acromion
- Supraspinatus tendon

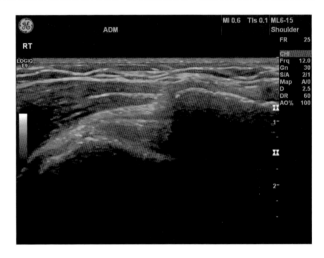

PATHOLOGY

● 1 *Rotator cuff pathology*

(a) Tears

(i) Full thickness tear

Tears are most common in the supraspinatus tendon, which roughly constitutes the anterior 1.5 cm of the cuff over the greater tuberosity. The tear may be classified on the basis of location as an anterior free edge, midsubstance or massive (when it extends across full width of supraspinatus and extends into infraspinatus).

Ultrasound features

- Tear extension from the articular to the bursal surface of the tendon
- Focal echo-poor defect, which may be filled with fluid
- Loss of normal superior convexity of the subacromial bursa and focal herniation of deltoid into the space created by tear
- Denudation of humeral head with deltoid directly overlying it
- Bony irregularity in the greater tuberosity at site of tear

(ii) Partial tears and tendinopathy

These account for approximately 15% of rotator cuff tears. It is difficult to differentiate partial thickness tears and tendinopathy on US, but as their clinical management is similar, much time should not be spent trying to differentiate between them. Partial tears may be classified as articular (more common) or bursal surface.

Ultrasound features

- Focal echo-poor area in at least two scan planes, which does not extend across full thickness of tendon
- Tendinopathy can be seen as heterogeneous echotexture of the tendon with associated tendon thickening

WHAT TO LOOK FOR

SCAN IMAGE

I (a)(i)

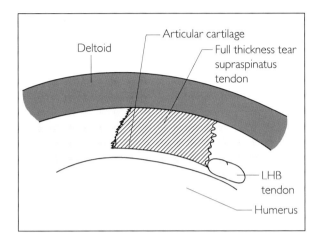

- Deltoid
- Articular cartilage
- Full thickness tear supraspinatus tendon
- LHB tendon
- Humerus

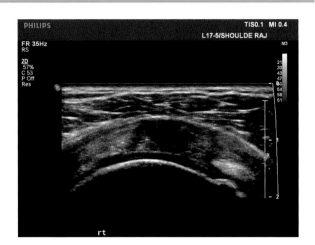

I (a)(ii)

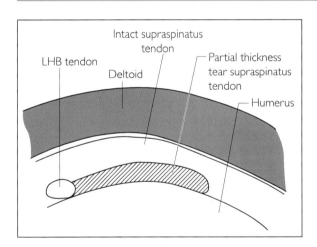

- Intact supraspinatus tendon
- LHB tendon
- Deltoid
- Partial thickness tear supraspinatus tendon
- Humerus

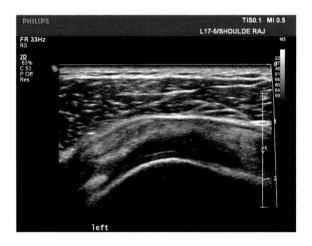

(b) Calcific tendinopathy

These are common findings affecting the rotator cuff tendons and consist of mainly hydroxyapatite deposition. The most common affected tendon is supraspinatus. Patients may be asymptomatic or present with acute or chronic pain.

Ultrasound features

- Intratendinous echo-bright foci that may be homogenously hyperechoic or may have associated acoustic shadowing (as seen with calculi in the abdomen)

● 2 Long head biceps tendon

(a) Disruption

LHB rupture is a clinical diagnosis associated with "Popeye sign" where swelling is noted in the anterior aspect of the mid arm. Tendon most commonly ruptures intra-articularly and myotendinous junction disruption is rare. LHB tears are often associated with rotator cuff tears involving supraspinatus and subscapularis tendons.

Ultrasound features

- Discontinuity of the tendon fibres
- Fluid and debris may be seen in the tendon sheath

WHAT TO LOOK FOR

SCAN IMAGE

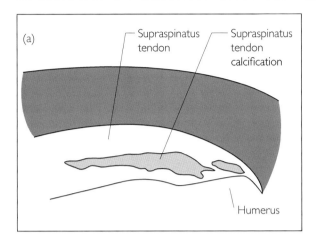

(a)
- Supraspinatus tendon
- Supraspinatus tendon calcification
- Humerus

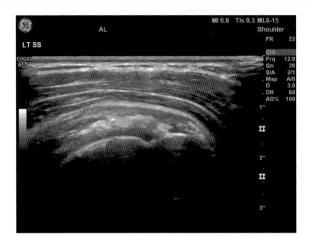

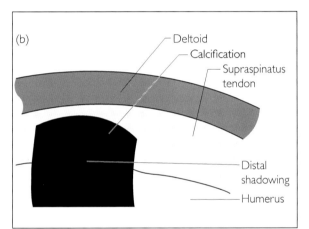

(b)
- Deltoid
- Calcification
- Supraspinatus tendon
- Distal shadowing
- Humerus

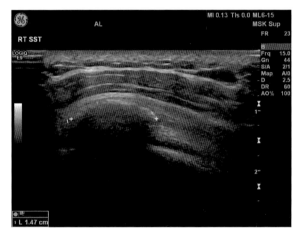

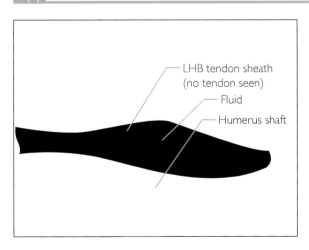

- LHB tendon sheath (no tendon seen)
- Fluid
- Humerus shaft

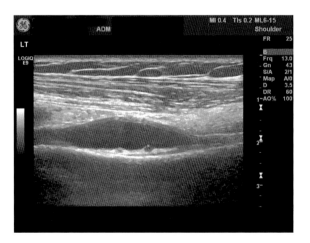

2(b)

(b) Tendinopathy

May occur due to chronic repetitive microtrauma and is more vulnerable due to its intra-articular course. Often occurs along with rotator cuff disease.

Ultrasound features
- Tendon thickening and heterogenecity
- Intrinsic tendon tears may be seen as echo-poor or echo-free areas

2(c)

(c) Tendon instability

LHB may migrate medially partially or completely (dislocation) out with the bicipital groove such that it may lie superficial or deep to the subscapularis tendon.

Ultrasound features
- Empty bicipital sulcus
- Tendon visualized medially over or under the subscapularis tendon

● 3 Subacromial subdeltoid bursal disease and impingement

3

Bursitis occurs in several shoulder disorders, the most common being impingement. Patients typically present with pain on shoulder abduction. Bursal effusion may also be present and should arouse suspicion of a full thickness rotator cuff tear, therefore careful examination of the tendon should be performed.

Ultrasound features
- Thickening of the synovial lining (echo-poor area) of the bursa
- Presence of fluid within the bursa, mainly in the dependent portion of the bursa, pooling along the lateral margin of greater tuberosity
- Dynamic examination for impingement demonstrates bunching of the bursa or ballottement of fluid lateral to the acromion

WHAT TO LOOK FOR

SCAN IMAGE

2(b)

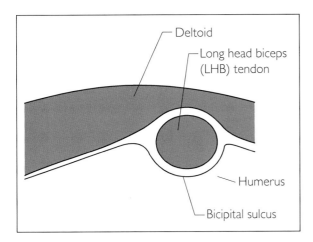

- Deltoid
- Long head biceps (LHB) tendon
- Humerus
- Bicipital sulcus

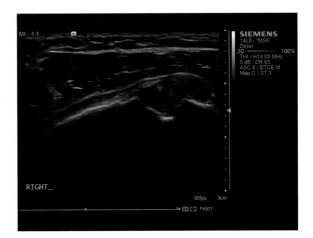

2(c)

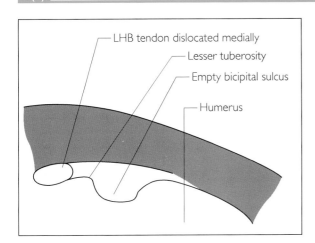

- LHB tendon dislocated medially
- Lesser tuberosity
- Empty bicipital sulcus
- Humerus

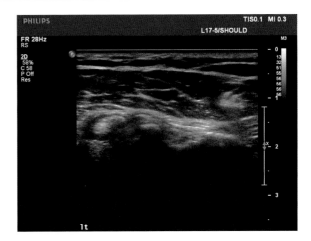

3

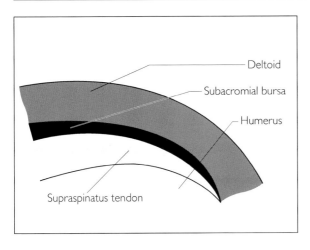

- Deltoid
- Subacromial bursa
- Humerus
- Supraspinatus tendon

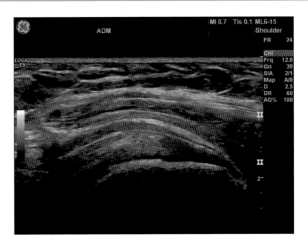

● 4 *Acromioclavicular joint pathology*

(a) Osteoarthritis

The acromioclavicular (AC) joint is a synovial joint prone to degenerative changes.

Ultrasound features

- Decrease in joint space, osteophyte formation, increased echo-poor changes in the joint and bulging of its capsule

(b) Subluxation/dislocation

Subluxation is due to AC joint ligamentous sprain and dislocation is the more severe injury, with additional disruption of the coracoclavicular ligament.

Ultrasound features

- Widening of the AC joint gap
- Increased echo-poor changes with thickening and oedema in the joint and capsule

(c) AC joint cyst (geyser phenomenon)

These present as painless masses overlying the AC joint, usually with an underlying rotator cuff tear.

Ultrasound features

- Cystic abnormality overlying the AC joint which may be multiseptated
- Look for rotator cuff tear

WHAT TO LOOK FOR

SCAN IMAGE

4(a)

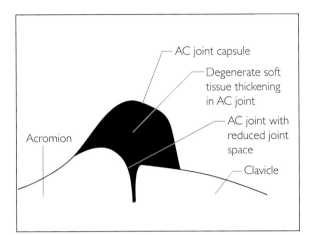

AC joint capsule

Degenerate soft tissue thickening in AC joint

AC joint with reduced joint space

Acromion

Clavicle

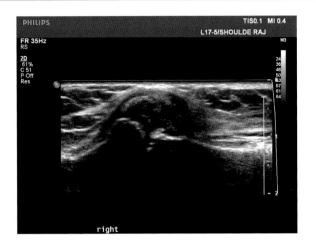

4(b)

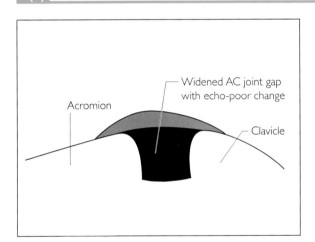

Widened AC joint gap with echo-poor change

Acromion

Clavicle

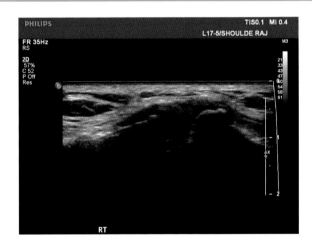

4(c)

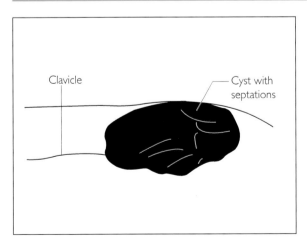

Clavicle

Cyst with septations

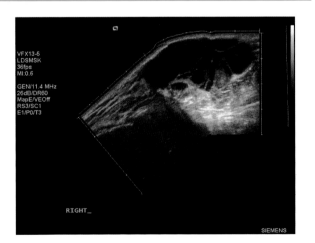

● 5 *Glenohumeral joint effusion*

US is a sensitive method for joint effusion; however, it cannot differentiate septic causes from other causes of joint effusion. Clinical correlation and analysis of joint fluid are required for definitive diagnosis.

Ultrasound features
- Fluid in the biceps tendon sheath that completely surrounds the tendon and extends across the length of the tendon
- Posterior aspect of joint examined in the longitudinal axis of infraspinatus demonstrating fluid in the joint and capsular bulging

● 6 *Adhesive capsulitis (Frozen shoulder)*

This is a self-limiting condition, which consists of reduced shoulder movements and pain. The first movement to be affected is external rotation and is one of the last to recover. More common in perimenopausal women, associated with diabetes, some drugs (e.g. isoniazide) and trauma..

Ultrasound features
- Relatively normal ultrasound examination with particular restriction of external rotation (making it difficult to obtain views of subscapularis tendon)
- Occasional findings of slightly increased fluid in the biceps tendon sheath and increased soft tissue echo-poor changes in anterior interval

WHAT TO LOOK FOR

SCAN IMAGE

5

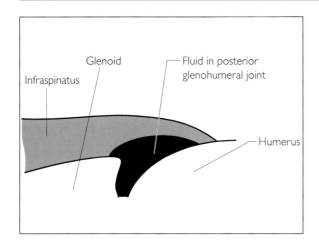

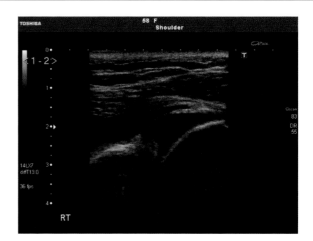

6

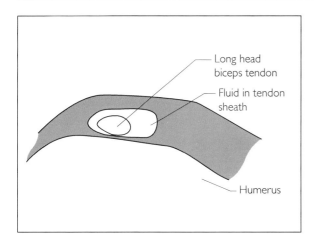

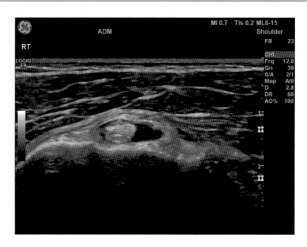

PERFORMING THE SCAN
● *Hip*

- **Patient position:** Supine.
- **Preparation:** None.
- **Probe:** High frequency (6–17 MHz) linear; in obese patients lower frequency probes can be used.
- **Machine:** Select from MSK settings; widescan or trapezoid FOV setting can be selected.
- **Method:** (a) The anterior aspect of the hip is examined for hip joint effusions or other pathologies; (b) the lateral aspect of the hip is examined for greater trochanteric bursal disease.

PROBE POSITION	INSTRUCTIONS

1

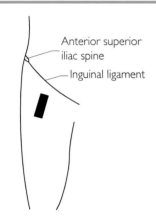

Anterior superior iliac spine

Inguinal ligament

- Examine the hip for joint effusion from the anterior aspect by placing the long axis of probe in a parasagittal plane and aligning it along the femoral neck. The anterior joint recess is well demonstrated as a concave bulging of the hyperechoic anterior capsule anterior to the femoral neck margin. The contralateral hip can be examined for any asymmetry of the joint capsule distension.

2

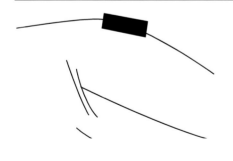

- Examine the hip for trochanteric bursal disease with the patient lying in a lateral position with the side to be examined lying superiorly. Place the probe longitudinally over the greater trochanter avoiding too much pressure and examine the posterolateral and posterior aspects of the greater trochanter. Over the anterior greater trochanter is the gluteus minimus tendon and lateral aspect hyperechoic band comprising the gluteus medius tendon. The posterolateral aspect of the greater trochanter the gluteus maximus tendon directly overlies the medius tendon. The bursae around the greater trochanter are not visible in normal individuals due to too small an amount of fluid.

WHAT TO LOOK FOR

SCAN IMAGE

1

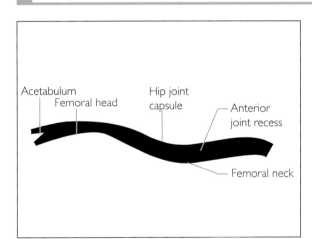

Acetabulum
Femoral head
Hip joint capsule
Anterior joint recess
Femoral neck

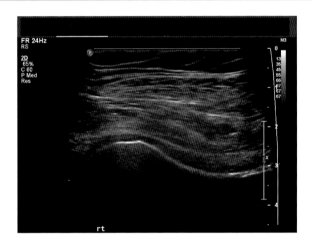

2

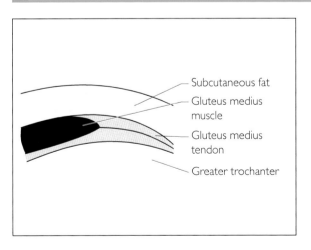

Subcutaneous fat
Gluteus medius muscle
Gluteus medius tendon
Greater trochanter

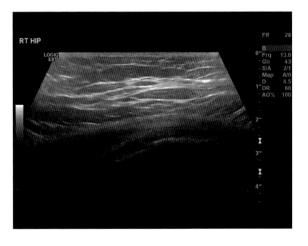

HIP PATHOLOGY

● 1 *Hip joint effusion*

1

This could be secondary to transient synovitis (seen in children), inflammatory causes or infection. Septic arthritis can have severe consequences and it is imperative to make an early diagnosis. Clinical and biochemical correlation is required and, if effusion is present, aspiration or surgical intervention would be necessary for definitive diagnosis.

Ultrasound features

- Bulging of the capsule at the anterior joint recess over the neck of the femur to a more convex rather than usual concave shape
- Increased echo-poor changes and/or fluid visualized in the recess
- Thickness of ≥7 mm of the anterior joint recess and/or difference of ≥2 mm between the recesses when compared with the contralateral joint

● 2 *Greater trochanteric bursitis*

2

Patients typically present with pain and tenderness on deep palpation over the lateral and posterolateral aspects of the greater trochanter. Middle-aged and elderly women are most commonly affected. The spectrum of findings includes bursitis, calcifications in the gluteus medius tendon or bursa and tendinopathy.

Ultrasound features

- Trochanteric bursa does not distend significantly with fluid and in cases of bursitis thickening or a thin rim of fluid is noted superficial to the gluteus medius tendon over the lateral and posterolateral greater trochanter deep to the gluteus maximus
- This area is also the target for US-guided steroid injections

WHAT TO LOOK FOR

SCAN IMAGE

1

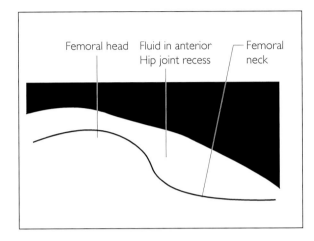

Femoral head   Fluid in anterior   Femoral
Hip joint recess   neck

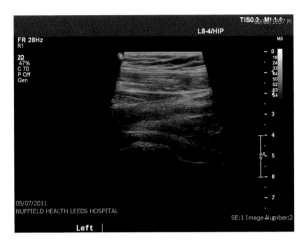

2

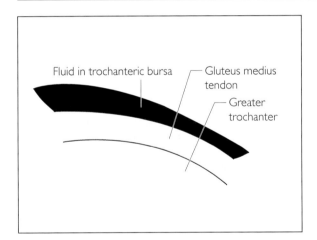

Fluid in trochanteric bursa   Gluteus medius
tendon
Greater
trochanter

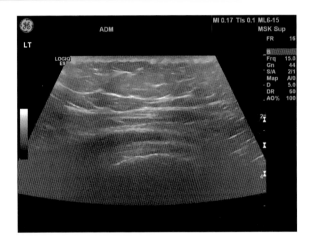

PERFORMING THE SCAN

● *Knee*

- Patient position: Supine.
- Preparation: None.
- Probe: High frequency (6–17 MHz) linear.
- Machine: Select the MSK setting.
- Method: The anterior knee is examined in a supine position with partial flexion (20–30°) at the knee, which can be obtained by keeping a pillow below the joint. This stretches the quadriceps and patellar tendons and enables their examination, removing any anisotropy seen in the extended state due to concave contour. The posterior knee is examined with the patient in a prone position and the popliteal fossa is examined in the transverse and sagittal planes.

PROBE POSITION	INSTRUCTIONS

1 Quadriceps tendon

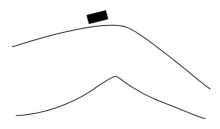

- Place the probe in the sagittal plane in the midline knee cranial to the patella such that the distal edge of the probe demonstrates the quadriceps insertion on the superior pole of the patella.
- Observe the multilayered fibrillar structure of the quadriceps tendon, which is formed by fusion of four tendons.
- Scan in longitudinal and transverse planes along the length of the tendon and cranially to the myotendinous junction region.

2 Patellar tendon

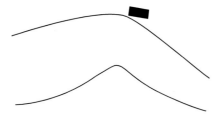

- Place the probe in midline directly over the patellar tendon and scan from its origin at the inferior pole of the patella to the distal insertion on the tibial tuberosity.
- Scan in both longitudinal and transverse planes and observe its thickness, uniform fibrillar structure, integrity and any prominent bursa deep to the distal insertion.

WHAT TO LOOK FOR

SCAN IMAGE

1 Quadriceps tendon

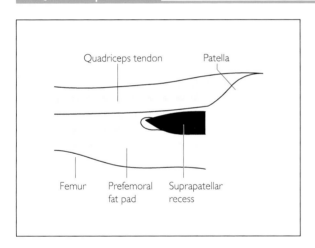

Quadriceps tendon   Patella

Femur   Prefemoral fat pad   Suprapatellar recess

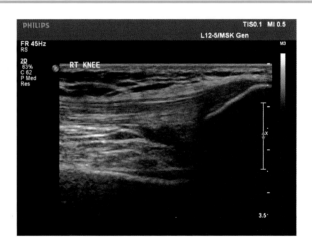

2 Patellar tendon

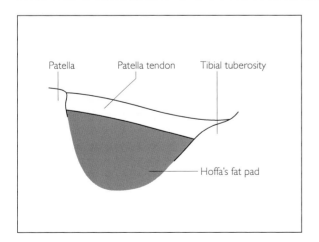

Patella   Patella tendon   Tibial tuberosity

Hoffa's fat pad

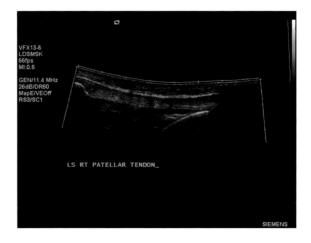

KNEE PATHOLOGY

● 1 Quadriceps tendon disruption

Most tears occur at or near the patellar attachment and clinically a gap may be palpated above the patella. Loss of active knee extension is the most consistent clinical finding. Aetiology includes trauma or secondary to underlying medical conditions such as SLE, rheumatoid arthritis and diabetes. Most tears are incomplete.

Ultrasound features
- Partial or full thickness loss of integrity of tendon
- Gap at tear site due to tendon retraction may be seen in complete tears
- In acute cases, haematoma and oedematous changes can be seen at tear site

● 2 Patellar tendon disease

Patellar tendinopathy occurs due to chronic overuse mainly in athletes involved in jumping such as basketball, volleyball and sprinting, hence the alternative name 'jumper's knee'. Patients usually present with anterior knee pain.

Ultrasound features
- Loss of normal fibrillar pattern with echo-poor changes and tendon thickening in the proximal central patellar tendon close to its origin
- Neovascularity demonstrated on colour or power Doppler

● 3 Baker's (popliteal) cyst

Arises as fluid-filled synovial lined outpouching from the posteromedial knee, characteristically arising from between the medial head of gastrocnemius and the semimembranosus tendon. Typically has 'speech bubble' configuration in the transverse plane. These are usually asymptomatic but may be palpable when large.

WHAT TO LOOK FOR

SCAN IMAGE

1

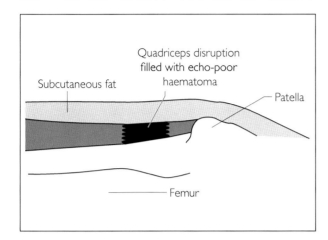

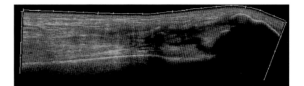

2

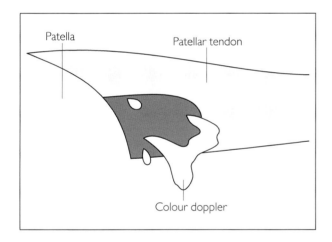

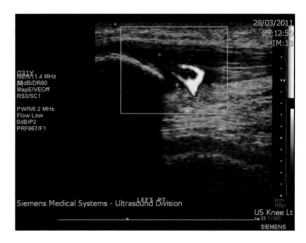

3

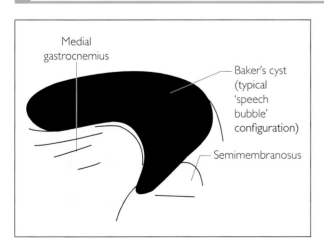

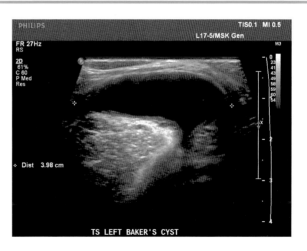

PERFORMING THE SCAN

● *Ankle and foot*

Achilles tendon

- **Patient position:** Prone.
- **Preparation:** None.
- **Probe**: High frequency (6–17 MHz) linear.
- **Machine**: Select the MSK setting.
- **Method**: The examination is performed with the patient lying prone and foot hanging beyond the examination table.

PROBE POSITION

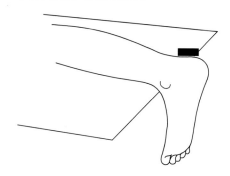

INSTRUCTIONS

- The probe is placed in the posterior midline distal leg in the sagittal and axial planes examining the tendon from the myotendinous junction to its insertion on the calcaneum.
- Examine the tendon for fibrillar pattern, thickness and integrity.
- Measure tendon dimensions in the anteroposterior plane while scanning transversely. Normal tendon thickness is 5–6 mm.

PATHOLOGY

● 1 *Achilles tendinopathy*

1

This is a common cause of heel pain and in the majority of cases is related to overuse activity such as running. Tendinopathy may be diffuse or focal and may be associated with tears. More commonly the proximal two-thirds of the tendon are affected.

Ultrasound features
- Diffuse or focal swelling (total tendon thickness >6 mm) of the tendon with echo-poor appearance
- Echo-free areas representing severe tendinosis or partial tears may be seen within the tendinopathic tendon
- Neovascularity seen on colour or power Doppler examination

WHAT TO LOOK FOR

SCAN IMAGE

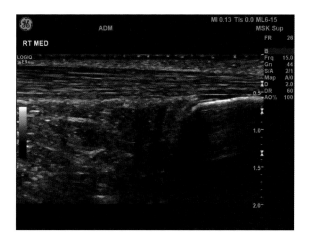

Achilles tendon   Retrocalcaneal buna

Kager's fat pad   Calcaneum

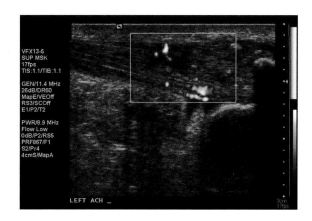

Insertional tendinopathy

Achilles tendon   Thickened tendon — Neovascularity

— Areas of calcification

— Calcaneum

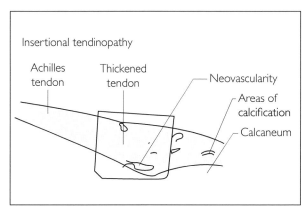

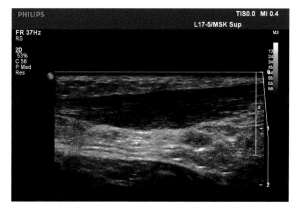

Non-insertional tendinopathy

Fusiform thickening mid Achilles tendon

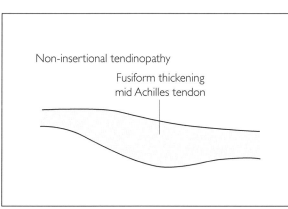

● 2 Achilles tendon rupture

Typically occurs in the third to fifth decade and is more common in men. Mostly from acute trauma, common causes being racket sports such as badminton. Previous tendinopathy predisposes to tendon rupture. The location of the rupture may be the mid region 2–6 cm proximal to calcaneal insertion (most common), at the myotendinous junction or avulsion of its attachment (least common). The tears may be partial or complete and it is important to state this in the report.

Ultrasound features

- Full thickness tear:
  - complete interruption or defect in the tendon, which is often filled with fluid and echo-poor haematoma in acute cases
  - dynamic examination should be performed whenever possible with plantar and dorsiflexion of foot looking for any increased gap at the tear site (this helps differentiate high grade partial from complete tear)
  - other signs are increased visualisation of plantaris tendon and posterior acoustic shadowing from the torn ends
- Partial thickness tear:
  - tear extends incompletely across the thickness of the tendon
  - dynamic examination as described above can help differentiate between high-grade partial and complete tears

WHAT TO LOOK FOR

SCAN IMAGE

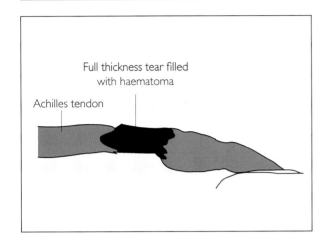

Full thickness tear filled with haematoma

Achilles tendon

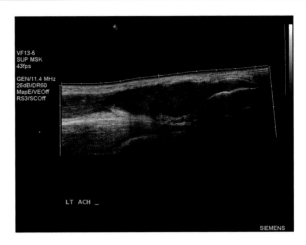

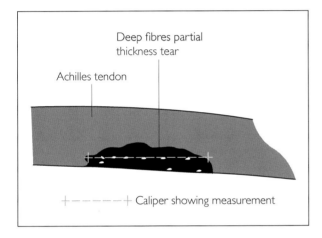

Deep fibres partial thickness tear

Achilles tendon

+ − − − − − + Caliper showing measurement

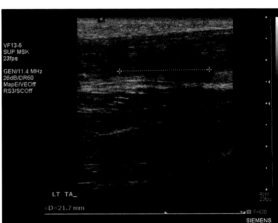

SOFT TISSUE MASSES

Soft tissue masses of the musculoskeletal system are extremely common. The vast majority are benign and the ratio of benign to malignant lesions is 1:100. Clinical history of recent/relatively rapid increase in size of lesion, presence of pain and underlying history of malignancy are symptoms that should raise suspicion for sarcoma. What the clinicians want to know is: (1) Is there a lesion? (2) Where is the lesion? and (3) What is the lesion?

High-resolution ultrasound and Doppler examination form the first-line investigation for most soft tissue masses. It also helps differentiate between pseudotumours (such as haematomas, cysts, abscess) and a true lesion. If a specific diagnosis cannot be provided and there is clinical concern, ultrasound can help guide percutaneous biopsy.

Soft tissue tumours are broadly classified according to the connective tissue they arise from: lipomatous, fibrous, nerve, fibrous, vascular, synovial and muscle.

Benign soft tissue tumours have more typical features allowing for a specific diagnosis. However, most sarcomas have similar appearances, typically having heterogeneous but predominantly echo-poor echotexture, deep location and avid internal vascularity with the presence of necrotic areas.

PERFORMING THE SCAN

- **Patient position:** Depends on the location of the soft tissue mass.
- **Preparation:** None.
- **Probe:** High frequency (6–17 MHz) linear.
- **Machine:** Select from MSK setting.
- **Method:** The aim is to fully visualize the mass to be able to give its anatomical location, echogenicity, size in three planes, any flow on Doppler, relationship(s) to important structures such as neurovascular bundles and try to give a definitive or differential diagnosis. If the lesion is large or long, an extended field of view is helpful in its assessment.

PATHOLOGY OF COMMON BENIGN SOFT TISSUE TUMOURS

● I Lipomatous tumours

Lipoma
This is the most common soft tissue tumour, and it can occur in almost any part of the body. Between 5% and 15% of patients can have multiple lipomas. Some lipomas do not have a capsule (unencapsulated) and can have thin (<2 mm) septa

Ultrasound features
- The typical subcutaneous lipoma is a well-defined, elliptical, compressible lesion having homogenous echo-bright echotexture and containing linear reflective striations running parallel to the skin
- May be superficial (subcutaneous) or deep (subfascial, muscle compartment)

Note: At times it may be impossible to differentiate between a benign lipoma and a well-differentiated liposarcoma on imaging alone. Current guidelines suggest that any lipomatous lesion over >5 cm and in a deep location should be referred to sarcoma specialists.

WHAT TO LOOK FOR

SCAN IMAGE

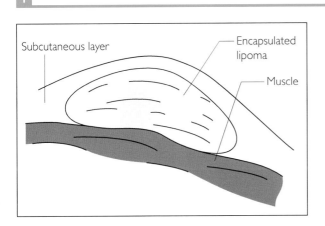

Subcutaneous layer

Encapsulated
lipoma

Muscle

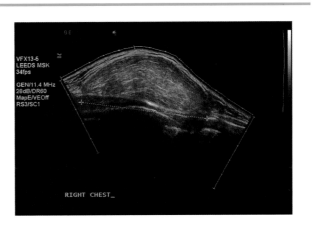

● 2 Vascular tumours

2

Haemangiomas and vascular malformations
These are common lesions that may be located in the skin, subcutaneous layer or muscle.

Ultrasound features
- Vascular malformations consist of tortuous and lacunar spaces with little intervening stroma, which is comparatively more in haemangiomas.

● 3 Nerve tumours

3

Neurofibromas and schwannomas
Often the clinical features will suggest the diagnosis such as history of neurofibromatosis or sharp shooting pain associated with the lesion.

Ultrasound features
- Well-circumscribed, and can sometimes be seen arising from the nerve
- Typically neurofibromas are located centrally and schwannomas eccentrically in the nerve, though this may not always be demonstrable
- Presence of colour or power Doppler flow

● 4 Fibrous tumours

4

Fibromatosis may be superficial or deep. Superficial fibromatosis may be palmar or plantar. In the palms, it leads to Duputyren's contracture and is a clinical diagnosis.

Plantar fibromatosis
Ultrasound features
- Echo-poor well-defined lesions related to the plantar fascia
- Larger lesions may be heterogeneous
- Sometimes may have blood flow on colour/power Doppler

Desmoid
Deep fibromatosis that occurs in the abdominal wall is called desmoid as illustrated in image opposite.

WHAT TO LOOK FOR

SCAN IMAGE

2

(a)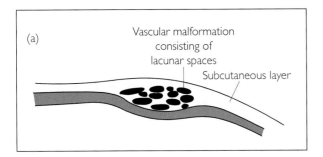

Vascular malformation
consisting of
lacunar spaces

Subcutaneous layer

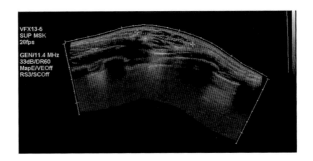

(b)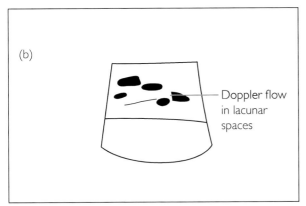

Doppler flow
in lacunar
spaces

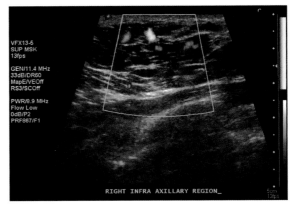

3

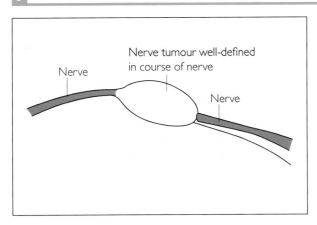

Nerve

Nerve tumour well-defined
in course of nerve

Nerve

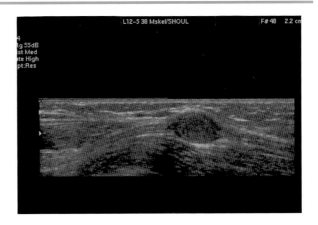

4

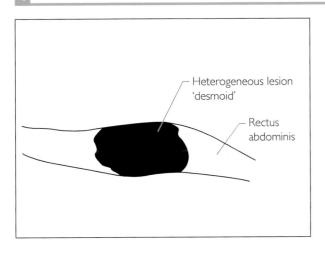

Heterogeneous lesion
'desmoid'

Rectus
abdominis

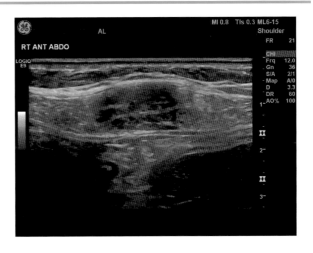

MALIGNANT SOFT TISSUE TUMOURS (SARCOMAS)

It is difficult to differentiate the subtype of sarcoma such as liposarcoma, malignant peripheral nerve sheath tumour (MPNST), fibrosarcoma, leiomyosarcoma or angiosarcoma on the basis of imaging. However, sarcomas have common features, which are as follows:

- Predominantly echo-poor appearances, sometimes heterogeneous nature
- Deep location
- Presence of blood flow on colour/power Doppler
- Necrotic areas
- Extension beyond one compartment

TUMOUR-LIKE LESIONS

● 1 *Haematoma*

1

Ultrasound features
- Variable ultrasound appearances ranging from echo-bright mass consisting of solid clot to echo-free liquefied abnormality

● 2 *Abscess*

2

Ultrasound features
- Echo-free purulent fluid collections that often have a capsule

WHAT TO LOOK FOR

SCAN IMAGE

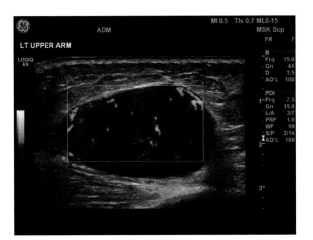

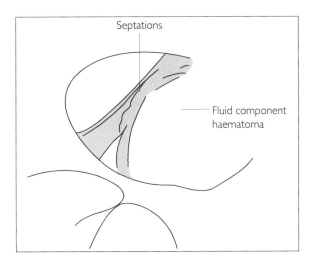

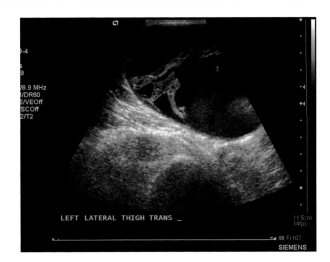

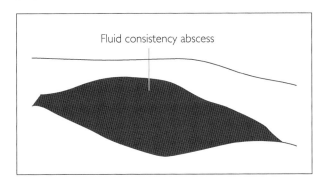

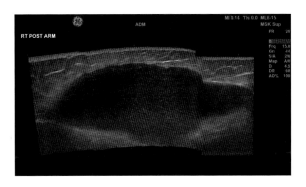

● *3 Sebaceous cyst*

3

Ultrasound features

- Well-defined lesions having internal echoes due to presence of keratin and lipid debris
- Typically occur in cutaneous location and have no internal vascularity on Doppler examination

● *4 Ganglion cyst*

4

Cystic lesion that has internal gelatinous content and arises from a joint or tendon. It is not always possible on imaging to demonstrate their origin from a tendon or joint.

Ultrasound features

- Well-defined cystic lesions that maybe multiseptated
- Arise close to joints and tendons

WHAT TO LOOK FOR

SCAN IMAGE

3

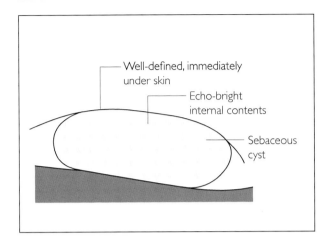

- Well-defined, immediately under skin
- Echo-bright internal contents
- Sebaceous cyst

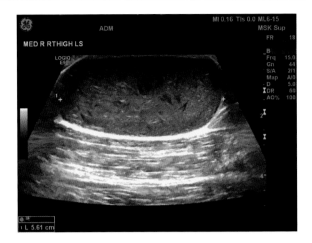

4

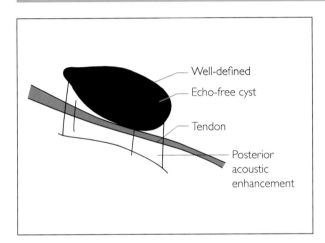

- Well-defined
- Echo-free cyst
- Tendon
- Posterior acoustic enhancement

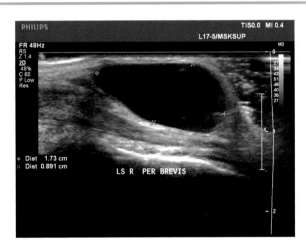

Index